connecting healthcare...

connecting healthcare...

IT TAKES A
VILLAGE
KEVIN PEREAU

TranscendIT Health,
Walnut Creek, CA

For Beth and Megan

ACKNOWLEDGMENTS

Above all, I want to express my love and gratitude to my wife Beth and my daughter Megan. Without their love and support, this book would never have happened.

I also would like to express profound gratitude to all the experts who contributed their views to this book, enriching it miles beyond what it could ever have been without them.

Thanks too to Alan Dino Hebel and his team at BookDesigners. com. They took some general ideas for what I wanted the design and the cover to be and turned them into a work of expressive and appropriate art.

I thank Barry Lenson, the editor who helped me turn a lot of ideas and plans into this book. We had fun and became good friends in the process. Thanks too to Varsana Tikovsky, a keen and insightful editor who proofread the manuscript and corrected a number of editorial issues that needed attention.

Last, I would like to thank you, my readers. In the pages ahead, you and I will enter an astonishing new world of connected care, an amazing and healthy journey we will take together.

Thank you for joining me, and welcome aboard!

Let's all plug in!

CONTENTS

FOREWORD

BY BRAD FLUEGEL

How is healthcare changing and who is benefitting? You are a consumer of healthcare services, and so am I. What plans should we be making and what do we need to be thinking about?

I approach those questions from the perspective that first of all, human beings don't live in the healthcare universe. They live in the real world. Even people who are dealing with diabetes or other chronic conditions are not exclusively focused on healthcare 24 hours a day. They are driving their cars to the grocery store or taking their kids to school.

In fact, most people are going to think only periodically about even chronic conditions. They have their lives to live. We have to meet them where they are and not force them to conform to the requirements of the healthcare system.

We do see that some wealthier people have the ability to devote more of their time, attention, and resources to managing their health and use expensive technologies. Unless you're a rich venture capitalist in Silicon Valley and can afford to be obsessed with all kinds of newfangled technologies that help you track fitness and health, chances are you won't. Most people don't have the time or money or energy.

I have noticed that the various stakeholders in the healthcare universe honestly care deeply about helping people. They do not only care about making a lot of money, even though many people in our society believe they do. The costs of insurance, prescription drugs, hospitals and physicians can be quite high, which reinforces that perception. Yet in my experience, most everyone in the world of healthcare is honestly trying to do good. They just don't know how to integrate into patients' lives and connect everything all together—their lives as both people and patients.

So, when I think about what the future holds for healthcare, I think we will see an integration of all the new technologies and data from various sources into people's lives on a moment-by-moment basis to support the goal of making lives and health better.

In practical terms, how will that be reached? I believe that, to engage consumers, everyone in healthcare needs to put a support system around consumers that interacts with them as part of their daily lives. We need to meet people where they are using tools, technologies and the places they are familiar with and already using.

That's a great place for digital health companies and retail organizations to play a role. One thing they can do is to develop technologies that can remotely monitor patients in their homes—in effect, to monitor how people are doing and alerting them and their care teams if a problem is detected.

Apple and many others are trying to do that with wearables, apps and other technologies. There are a whole slew of other companies, some of which are profiled in this book, that are trying to use technology supported by services to help people live healthier lives and better manage their chronic conditions.

Retailers are also diving deep into this. We have to remember that although customers are going online more and more, they still go to stores a lot. That is not going away. So companies like Walgreens and CVS are creating what CVS calls health hubs and what Walgreens calls health destinations within some of their stores. In them, people can now meet with a clinician for urgent issues, as well as for more chronic concerns, get lab tests, discuss their diets and get other services as well.

But at the end of the day, retailers and technology companies can't do it all by themselves. Traditional players have to lead on this as well. Doctors and health systems will continue to have an important role to play, because they're still most trusted by the patients who are under their care. And so some of the tools, whether they are services from retailers or technology companies, will need to be integrated with the services that physicians are providing to their patients, so that these newer telehealth and digital services don't sit on an island that is disconnected from the regular care pathways that many patients might be on. Patients often look to and trust their primary care providers and specialist physicians, and that will not change.

We have seen that happen during Covid-19. To be sure the pandemic brought about a lot of change in healthcare, but one of the things that I found most interesting was that although there was a big spike in telehealth visits to telehealth providers, there was also a massive increase in the telehealth offerings from traditional providers—people still wanted to interact with physicians they knew and trusted. Telehealth did not cause people to turn away from that. They still wanted to have a relationship with someone, often their doctor, or with someone in their doctor's practice. They didn't want to get advice or care from some random doctor, or some technology portal other than perhaps for some kind of kind of acute issue that emerged. The acceptance of telehealth from traditional providers was the real game-changer and will open the door to more convenient care for patients and improve outcomes. They will need technology to help them connect it all.

Another important change during the pandemic was that there came to be reimbursement parity between online and in-person visits. Whether you saw your physician during a telemedicine session or in his or her office, the provider received the same amount of money. That drove a massive cultural shift within providers that I think is going to stick. I believe that in the long term that change will be better for patients. Telemedicine is not going to replace in-person visits. But I think it represents a step change in usage for the traditional systems.

The fact that more people were working remotely during the

pandemic brought about change in employer-provided programs too. There were suddenly more employees working from home, sometimes part-time, and often with children at home too. This led to stress that was exacerbated by the isolation and loneliness that accompanied the lockdowns. Mental health issues and access to care became issues that employers and health plans had to address. Here again technology and connection have an important role to play.

Yet it is surprising that during the pandemic, the overall number of mental health visits came down—virtual visits were way up but more than offset by the decline in physical visits. I think that's going to create a big crisis, particularly for kids. The prevalence of eating disorders and anxiety and depression among young people who haven't been able to go to school or be socialized is a concern. There could be a huge wave of adverse events just waiting to happen down the road. That's something the industry has to anticipate and find ways to fix.

I'm also concerned that preventive screenings and care delayed during the pandemic may lead to a spike in illnesses and costs over the longer term. Technologies like those described in this book will be critical to addressing all of these issues.

And then lastly, I'd say with regard to health plans, they're all trying to get closer to patients and closer to their members. And I think they'll continue to do that. Over time, they will stitch together a system across not just traditional healthcare providers, but technologies, non-traditional business partners and others that are interacting with their members. They have an important navigational role to play in the future healthcare system. That's not possible without the connectedness advocated in this book.

So, what does all this innovation mean? Not much if you don't connect to it, which is what this book explores. It has been said that our smartphones are democratizing healthcare in much the same way that Gutenberg's printing press did the written word back in the 14th century. While regulation has slowly caught up to how to better integrate new technologies into our reimbursement workflows, *It Takes a Village* explains how you can tap in to take advantage and take control of your health. There is a cornucopia of resources available to you today that you never had before. You can't benefit unless you plug in and get connected. All you need is your smartphone. To your health!

ABOUT BRAD FLUEGEL

Brad Fluegel currently advises healthcare organizations, entrepreneurs, private equity firms and other participants in healthcare. He recently retired from being the Senior Vice President and Chief Strategy Officer at Walgreens based in Deerfield, IL.

Brad now serves on the Board of Directors at Metropolitan Jewish Health System in New York City, Performant Financial Corporation, Premera Blue Cross and Alight Solutions. He served on the board of Fitbit until its sale to Google in early 2021.

Brad earned a master's degree in public policy from Harvard University's Kennedy School of Government and a Bachelor of Arts in business administration from the University of Washington. He also serves as a lecturer at the University of Pennsylvania's Wharton School of Business.

INTRODUCTION

Welcome to *It Takes a Village*—the continuing story of how healthcare technology is better connecting you with all the resources you need to get and stay healthy. Since the Affordable Care Act was first enacted, we have seen an amazing technology explosion in healthcare. Over the last 10 years, we have made monumental strides in improving how we manage populations of health and creating a more consumer-like healthcare experience. We have broken down barriers and moved the needle in improving the health of our nation. We have also learned that technology alone won't be enough to help us fix our healthcare crisis. As consumers of healthcare services, what will it take and what role can we play? Increasingly, the impetus for disruption and change is coming from the most unlikely of places: consumers!

My first book *The Digital Health Revolution*, focused on how our smart phones are changing the way you and I manage our health by better connecting us to our stakeholders in healthcare. Our smartphones have democratized healthcare the way Gutenberg's printing press democratized the written word back in the 14ᵗʰ century. Patients are better involved in their recoveries because they are better informed and better connected. As the focus shifts from chronic care management to simply staying healthy, staying connected has never been easier and more important.

For this book, I interviewed 30 of healthcare's top thought leaders. I caught up with who is innovating and how end-users can take advantage. We provide you with examples of how people with diabetes can now capture and share their blood values with their doctors while digital health tools help supply them with tips and tricks for managing their condition. These same principles can be applied to literally any population of health, including those who are trying to avoid that trip to the doctor in the first place. There were many epiphanies along the way, but the final summation is that we are now on the cusp of connected health where all of our health data is actionable. Simply said, expectations are changing. If we share our personal health data, it is because we expect an immediate benefit in return.

Actionable health data and a connected world are fascinating new concepts. *It Takes a Village* explores how digital health technologies are now extending what we have long thought of as healthcare and begs the question, what else needs to connect? We again feature insights from some of healthcare's biggest names and thought leaders. From the emergence of retail health to everyday nutrition and fitness. We are also discovering that better managing the social determinants of health (SDOH) means activating and connecting schools, mental health facilities, recovery centers and gyms. It can't happen without our participation and connecting has never been easier.

WHAT MOTIVATED ME TO WRITE THIS BOOK?

I was driven to start writing about healthcare after reconnecting with a couple of schoolmates in Vermont where I grew up. Both confided in me that they now have type 2 diabetes. Neither was remotely aware of the tools and devices that are now available for tracking, analyzing and better connecting them with the people who can help them thrive with their diabetes. I thought, what good is Virta Health (which has reversed diabetes in more than 50,000 patients) if nobody has ever heard of them? So much innovation has happened over the last ten years, it is time we all catch up. Healthcare companies of all kinds have been busy innovating and investing in solutions that are easy to use and integrated into your providers' infrastructure capabilities as well as your Health Savings Account and Apple Health.

Health is the new wealth – it always has been - and it is a non-traditional group of new players who are emerging to help us get and stay healthy. Imagine walking into your local retail pharmacy to pick up a prescription. You have some time to kill so you wander over to their clinic where you spend a few moments talking to a nutritionist about the best foods that people with diabetes should avoid and what foods to embrace. Together, you build out a meal plan for the week. Each day, your meals are delivered right to your door by your local grocer. You are already using smart scales to capture your weight, BMI, and body fat. Couple that with your glucose readings, activity trackers and the meals you log every day, and you get a sense that not only can you manage your chronically monitored condition, but you can thrive with it or maybe even reverse it. Your provider now has a holistic look at how your diet and lifestyle come together to affect your health. You now have a better understanding of cause and effect and how our daily choices all add up to make a difference. You also have the tools for how to make better decisions. We are developing longitudinal relationships and better understanding of what drives poor health.

What are some of our lessons learned from this wave of digital health innovation? Much of what we do in healthcare focuses on our symptoms, but not the root causes of our problems. An eye-popping example of this is California's Surgeon General Nadine Burke Harris's realization that social determinants of health (SDOH) and adverse childhood experiences (ACE) are a huge contributor to poor health and require more than a doctor and a set of tech tools to manage. Because of that, we have included sensational input from Stevon Cook, Commissioner of the San Francisco Board of Education, and Austin Buettner from the Los Angeles Unified School District, on the roles that schools can play in ensuring the health of our students. Will it surprise anyone if mental health and social workers become an important everyday resource for students, or become an integral part of your local school or pharmacy? As former CMS Director and Board Member at United States of Care and Townhall Ventures Andy Slavitt likes to say, "Healthy kids make for healthier adults."

HEALTHCARE VS. SICK CARE

The term healthcare in itself is a bit of a misnomer. In reality, it has always been about sick care. We need to turn the corner and start focusing on how to get and stay healthy. My first healthcare company begged the question: what is good health? At its very core, it is a combination of who we are (our biometrics), what we do (our activities) and how we feel (our mental state of mind). In this book we will explore who is doing what to help us manage all three.

Perhaps the most exciting dynamic we have seen is the rise of retail health and the surge of new entrants into this space. The big data explosion is now transitioning us from backwards-looking analysis at what just happened to a forward-looking view at what we can do about preventing health problems in the first place. We now expect our health data to be actionable and we expect to be able to share our personal data with trusted sources who can help us stay healthy. Increasingly, those trusted sources are innovators who are already working with our providers and insurers. Nobody pulls that together quite like our local pharmacy.

When we first started writing *It Takes a Village,* we didn't anticipate we would be working through a pandemic. Who could have anticipated that? Because of that, we checked in with Peter Lee of Covered California and Kevin Mullin from the Green Mountain Care Board in Vermont to see how anyone losing their employer-provided benefits due to the downturn in the economy could continue their healthcare benefits. We also explored how providers are responding to the challenge with solutions that keep us connected to all the resources we need in health-care, whether we have COVID-19 or not. Who better than the American Telehealth Association and Bright.md to weigh in with their insights?

Perhaps the biggest take-away from all of our discussions was a subtle one. It isn't enough to connect us better within health-care. We need to also connect and recognize the interdependencies that drive health problems in the first place. If our children atrophy at school because they don't exercise and eat right, how can we later expect healthcare to fix the problems we are unwittingly creating?

This book is for you. Get caught up and get connected.

CHAPTER ONE
HARVESTING LESSONS LEARNED

If you have read my first book *The Digital Healthcare Revolution*, I want to welcome you back. If you haven't read that book, you will not miss a beat in exploring how you can benefit from digital health in the pages ahead.

As you know, technology doesn't stop innovating—ever. And the innovators don't stop trying to develop technologies that solve problems. So here we are again, exploring healthcare, one of the timeliest topics anywhere.

As we look back on the last 10 years, I believe there are some realities we can agree on. We know that this time has certainly been disruptive. Healthcare regulation, and the increased levels of investment that it spurred have exerted a profound effect on how health plans, payers, and providers service your needs. And more importantly, on how they interact with us. To boil it all down, they have become more accessible than ever before.

We can now connect with greater ease to our healthcare providers and clinicians and other stakeholders within healthcare that can help us live life to the fullest. And increasingly, we can do that without even going in to see a doctor.

AN AGE OF HEALTHY CURIOSITY

All these changes have awakened people's curiosity about their own health and engaged them in learning how to best manage their health to stay fit and healthy.

This change didn't just happen because staying fit and healthy is fun to do, but it's easy to get addicted to the endorphin rush of tracking what happens during a workout. We have discovered the rewarding processes of how tracking our BMI, body fat, weight, blood pressure, cholesterol, and other data can be used for our benefit in a variety of ways.

There aren't enough gadgets for some people who belong in the fit and healthy category. That said some of us are monitoring to manage ongoing or chronic conditions. We might require a persistent nudge or device to track something, or a clinician to help stay the course and learn how to thrive with our condition.

For people who are fit and healthy, we've made great strides. But to help us understand better what else is taking place, let's revisit some lessons learned from my last book *The Digital Healthcare Revolution.*

THREE PHASES OF DIGITAL HEALTHCARE

Digital Health 1.0, 2011- 2014

This was the time when we dispelled the popular myth that people wouldn't engage in, much less care about, their health. You would frequently hear healthcare executives say, "We can't get members or patients to engage when it comes to their own health." We saw the flaws in this thinking when thousands of healthcare apps appeared overnight, and new marketplaces flourished. The first wave of health tech innovation designed from the ground up to treat healthcare like a shopping experience came from outside of the industry and the data was designed to be share-able.

"We just can't get people to engage" is now yesterday's battle cry. If anything, there seems to be a growing appetite among consumers to become more involved in their healthcare. Consumers are donning Fitbits, buying bathroom scales that keep ongoing data about their daily weigh-ins, and taking other steps to gather and monitor their data.

People became more engaged in their own healthcare and wellbeing. This explosion of digital health apps dispels the popular myth that people won't engage, share or be held accountable. We had never given them tools like this before and they couldn't download these new healthcare apps fast enough.

Digital Health 2.0 2014-2019

The app explosion soon gave way to the platform explosion. Big data was the new battle cry. You sometimes hear this described as the quantified self movement—a time when people warmed to the idea of using devices to track just about everything. The smartest people in the room could look backwards and tell you what just happened and why. We even got good about predicting what would happen next.

Digital Health 3.0, 2020 - present

I like to call this period, connected health. When I wrote *The Digital Health Revolution*, we were only on the cusp. Now, we are living it. Consumers are fully engaged and collecting data that is being fed to analytics platforms that help us decide what to do next. The focus has shifted from understanding what just happened to how to manage to better outcomes. We are making our data actionable by connecting it to the stakeholders who help keep us healthy and leveraging their keen insights. We are working with coordinated care teams who use the data captured by digital health assets to keep us well, not treat us after we become ill.

Historically, healthcare has been about treating people when they are sick, with not much emphasis on keeping them healthy. But that is now changing.

The myth that people won't engage in their health and wellness has now been absolutely obliterated. People have embraced Google Fit, Apple Health, and many other tools because it is as easy as turning on their smartphones. The adoption was so sudden and so widespread that it caught many in the industry by surprise. From health plans to providers, nobody expected people to dig in and sustain engagement at this level.

We've learned a lot about people and what motivates them, and they do want to be healthy. Curiosity was definitely a driver. Suddenly we started measuring everything. The quantified self movement has given way to connected health and actionable data, and we can't generate enough data about our own personal health fast enough.

Increasingly, we are doing this in near real time. If you're a patient monitoring a chronic condition and you have multiple stakeholders helping you monitor your condition, it is no longer a shock to you that the clinicians, nurses and doctors within your provider network will all have access to the same data while being able to take action at the appropriate time to help you.

But at the same time, are we addressing the root cause of what's causing poor health in the first place, or simply taking care of problems as we see them arise? We have spent much of the past decade connecting everything within healthcare.

And I think that it's time to ask a question, and it's a simple one . . .

What needs to connect to healthcare that isn't connected now?

What are the drivers for the health problems we are facing? We realize that there are factors that cause stress. There are factors that cause diabetes. There are factors that cause hypertension and heart problems.

Typically, those factors are things that we do to ourselves, like lifestyle choices, but not always.

The take-away is getting healthier needs to be a participator sport. It is something in which we can all take an active role. But the process can be made more efficient when we take steps like aligning incentives for providers and changing reimbursement models.

We can only do so much with technology alone. At the end of the day, it really does take a village. It takes everyone rowing in the same direction.

That is what we will be exploring in this book:

Chapter Two will introduce us to some of the people who are driving innovation.

Chapter Three will let us hear from some of "the new disruptors" in the world of healthcare.

Chapter Four is about the role that nutrition is playing in the healthcare revolution.

Chapter Five will explore how schools are connecting to the world of healthcare.

Chapter Six will take us into the state of reform in healthcare.

Chapter Seven will be about life hacks and the role they play.

Chapter Eight will take us through the pandemic and explore the role that payers and providers have played, and how they have changed.

Chapter Nine will recap, telling us where healthcare has been so far, and make some predictions where we are going next.

MEET TWO INNOVATORS

Omada Health and Virta Health are two companies that are at the forefront of what is happening in our village – for the inventive ways they are using data to help patients better manage type 2 diabetes. That, we know, represents one of the loftiest challenges on the healthcare landscape—for people who suffer from the disease, to care providers, to payers, to insurance companies. In short, to everyone who is located anywhere in the world of healthcare.

What are these two companies doing to reshape the way we are dealing with this disease, which has reached pandemic proportions around the world?

Omada Health was founded in 2011 to offer a new way to help people with prediabetes reduce their risk of developing type 2 diabetes, and to help people who already have type 2 diabetes manage their disease more effectively. Today, upwards of 200,000 people are using Omada to lead much more healthy lives.

How do people sign up for the Omada program? You begin by visiting the Omada website, where you answer questions to find out whether you are at risk for chronic disease. If you are, you qualify to join Omada. A short time later, an Omada digital scale arrives in a box. It looks much like any other digital bathroom scale, but it contains a cellular device that communicates with the Omada care team and feeds data to the participant's private profile.

That begins the process, which moves through two distinct phases of care. During the first phase—called Foundations—members get to know themselves better by tracking and submitting their weight, food, activity, and other data. They do so as part of a small group setting and they work with an Omada coach who gives advice on how they are managing their care, and what could be improved. After the first phase, they switch to Focus, where they are coached and supported on hyper-personalized goals based on their progress in Foundations as they make their healthy new habits part of their lives.

The Omada program works. Within the first year of participation, Omada members consistently lose significant amounts of weight. People who are pre-diabetic lose the amount of weight associated with a 30 percent reduction in the risk of developing type 2 diabetes, a 16 percent reduction in the risk of stroke, and a 13 percent reduction in the risk of heart disease. Those are verified statistics, because Omada conducts ongoing clinical studies of members' health.

Virta Health, another remarkable innovator in the care of diabetes type 2, makes a lofty claim that it can back up with statistics. The company maintains that it has reversed type 2 diabetes in more than 50,000 of the company's members.

That is amazing, when you consider where we were only five years ago—when anyone who claimed to have "reversed" diabetes was sure to become the object of skepticism, or worse.

After joining Virta Health and answering some screening questions, a new member receives a welcome kit that includes a "smart" connected blood glucose meter, test strips, a smart scale, and other supplies. That member is then assigned a team of monitors and care providers that includes a care coach, a physician-led team of medical specialists, educational resources that include diet and nutritional planning, as well as connections to a community of other Virta Health members who are also engaged in the process of controlling—and even reversing—their diabetes.

Both Omada and Virta provide a new generation of seamless care that cuts across the boundaries of nutrition, primary care, specialist care, exercise, and more. They are doing more than just gathering data, they are using that data to provide care and counseling in a frictionless way. Increasingly, they are taking action on your health data in near real time.

And although we will meet Jenny Craig again several times later in this book, let me mention it in this chapter because this weight loss/nutritional counseling company is at the forefront of designing and delivering care to people who would like to lose weight and improve their intake of healthful foods.

How is Jenny Craig moving the needle in the universe of nutrition and weight loss? Gathering and evaluating individual data is part of the process. But the company is forging new kinds of category-cutting business deals that are poised to cause notable changes in both the weight loss and healthcare industries.

Jenny Craig nutritional counselors can already be found in many Walgreens pharmacies and will soon be found in more. Note too that Walgreens is moving to provide primary care medical services. Plus, increasing cooperation between Jenny Craig, Walgreens and Krogers grocery stores promises a new way to integrate nutrition and meal preparation with pharmacy and even primary medical care.

Integrations like these are becoming the new normal and Walgreens is setting the standard.

CHAPTER TWO

WHO IS DRIVING
THE INNOVATION?

Who is driving the innovation that we are seeing in healthcare?

What are those companies doing?

Why are these changes happening now?

Although those might be simple questions, finding the answers is complex. Arguably, healthcare has been badly broken for decades. Even when it is easy to see what needs to be changed, the process of fixing things is complex, multi-faceted, expensive, and the industry has been resistant to change. These problems are entrenched. And when that is the case, it can be difficult to understand what exactly is taking place right before our eyes.

So, how do you boil the ocean? The answer is one cup at a time. You start by focusing on solving real-world problems and then building incrementally from there. If you think about where we were ten short years ago and where we are now, you realize a couple of things about healthcare. One, many of our problems are self-inflicted. Two, perfect should never be the enemy of improvement. Early on, the pushback to some of the digital health innovations were mind-numbing. The naysayers are still out there but let's keep everything in perspective. The most important metric we can track in healthcare is better outcomes. Reducing cost is absolutely important but arguably, don't better outcomes do just that?

We can't really improve the health of our nation without accepting some common goals and knowing how to achieve them. Let's meet some of the drivers of all the disruption.

MEET ROCK HEALTH

Rock Health is an early-stage digital health venture fund and advisory services firm with headquarters in San Francisco. Rock Health states that it is the first venture fund dedicated to digital health. Its large and growing portfolio includes some of the most innovative healthcare companies in segments that include dental benefits management, telehealth, HIPAA compliance, pediatric care management, predictive analytics, and prescription and pharmaceuticals management. I've watched Rock Health progress from being an idea to being an incubator, a concept accelerator and now, a full-service seed capital fund and healthcare research center. The significance of that to consumers is simply that this company has evolved in amazing ways and negotiated their pivots while driving much of the change we need in healthcare.

Earlier in its life, Rock Health was instrumental in bringing together innovators and advisors to simply get good ideas off the ground. They sought out early-stage thinkers unwilling to accept healthcare's entrenched thinking. They challenged norms and they challenged innovators. They asked tough questions coming right out of the gates.

- How does your solution solve a real-world healthcare problem?
- Who is on point for managing the problem?

I am constantly on their website and today, I see that they're branching into social activism. They have recently released a report about diversity, or the lack thereof, in healthcare. And they're quick to call out not only the lack of minority-led businesses, but the lack of minorities in the C-suite level at many of our industry's leading organizations.

They have over 70 portfolio companies, and that number is growing. They have focused on stoking innovation to better manage entire populations of health as well as challenging us to address the gaps we still have around social determinants of health (SDOH), mental health and addiction afflictions. We checked in recently with Megan Zweig, one of the brightest minds in healthcare and an up-and-coming thought leader who is increasingly being sought out for her perspective by healthcare conferences.

MEGAN ZWEIG OF ROCK HEALTH
ON CULTIVATING INNOVATION IN HEALTHCARE
Megan Zweig is Chief Operating Officer of Rock Health.

"I think one of the ways in which Rock Health has evolved is thinking about the value proposition that we bring to the ecosystem," says Megan. "When we were founded, the intention was to equip tech entrepreneurs to create great products in the highly complex, regulated space of healthcare. That value proposition has evolved because we recognized that there can be a huge gap between the startup healthcare innovators and their buyers or the doctors on the enterprise side of the market. And so instead of exclusively focusing on Rock Health providing the capital to support those entrepreneurs, we decided that it was important to build the second arm of our business, our advisory services, by offering research, support, insights, and consulting support to healthcare enterprises that are thinking about their digital transformation. Our goal is to leverage the tools and solutions that our portfolio companies have developed and help get them to market where we believe they can make a real difference.

"At Rock Health, we really think about ourselves as overcoming the friction that can exist between startups and enterprise. And we support both sides, whether through our fund on the startup side or through our advisory services where we partner with enterprise healthcare."

Anyone who has dared wade into healthcare can tell you about friction. Healthcare remains one of the most complex industries in the world and frequently, even the best ideas atrophy for lack of traction. That is where Rock Health comes in.

ROCK HEALTH'S LEVELS OF INVOLVEMENT

As a venture fund, Rock Health works with pharma companies, health systems and health plans. But Megan stresses that the underlying philosophy is what she calls "a holistic approach to caring for patients." This is incredibly important because wherever you are in healthcare's value chain, getting patients to a better outcome is the holy grail.

"We believe that physical and mental health and wellbeing are all intertwined, even though in the past they have been siloed," Megan explains. "I think we're seeing more digital companies recognize that if they are trying to encourage behavior change and healthier habits, they also have to address some of the mental issues that might be getting in the way of forming healthy habits." In essence, you can't expect technology alone to fix things, you need to develop solutions that encourage better and more educated participation.

That makes sense—but it represents a way of thinking that many companies in healthcare have been slow to adopt. It seems so obvious! In the past, a lot of companies believed that if they could get patients to organize their pill boxes, they would, of course, take their medications. We now know they didn't. And the reasons why are becoming increasingly clear. Many are depressed, maybe even denying that they are dealing with a condition that they have to take control of; or family or other issues take a higher priority than dealing with their own health problems right now. Some are overwhelmed with feelings of hopelessness. Sure, we all want to eat better but healthy foods typically cost us more. How can you argue with a $5 Happy Meal that leaves you feeling full but absolutely puts you on the obesity track?

Since traditional approaches have not been working, Rock Health is encouraging companies to expand the scope of how they are thinking about and interacting with customers. One approach that Megan cites is saying to consumers, "We're going to give you a chunk of money that you'll start out with. But if you don't follow through on your medication regimen, we're going to take some of that money away each time you don't fulfill your goal."

That's actually highly motivating to people. And we are finding that this sort of motivation works, even with populations that are difficult to engage. In essence, Rock Health is probing more into the psychology of what makes people tick. They are drilling down to the root causes of what drives poor health and what can we do about it. Why do we keep making bad decisions?

Another point of resistance that is not unique to the customers who are served by the companies Rock Health has helped is the fact that most people are comfortable sharing data with their physician, but not yet comfortable sharing with their health plan. That tendency steadily declines when people are asked to share their health data with the government, with tech companies and with other stakeholders in healthcare. Curiously, that resistance to sharing has grown even more acute during the Covid-19 pandemic, even though you might reasonably have come to expect that the opposite would have happened.

ON ACCESSING THE DIGITAL "FRONT DOOR"

The concept of the digital front door has become a popular talking point in the age of Covid-19. In brief, it is a term that refers to the point of entry where healthcare consumers first begin to digitally engage with those who can help them understand and manage their health-related conditions.

"The way that we at Rock Health think about the digital front door is relatively simple," Megan explains. "It's the point at which you decide that something's up with your health, and you want to use technology to access some sort of care or treatment for that particular issue.

"The steps people take at that point are different. Maybe I'm just talking to my partner about what's up with my health. And then maybe we decide to Google it just to see what do these symptoms mean? And then maybe we kind of understand where this condition or problem might be going, and we want to talk to a provider, or schedule an appointment to talk to an expert. We also have to figure out whom we want to see and where we want to go, is it covered by my health plan and are they in my network? How close are they to where I live? Have I been to them before? Do they look friendly based on their Yelp reviews?" Most people expect to be able to access all this from their smartphone. Who would have ever thought only a few short years ago that your healthcare provider would be concerned about their Yelp scores? Consumerizing our healthcare experience means being able to shop for what we need, seeing how others rate that service and then scheduling and paying for all this while integrated into easy-to-navigate screens. Add to this the convergence of data from our favorite devices and compelling timely content and you have the recipe for better managing entire populations of health. One such population is people with diabetes. This should not be a life defining or restricting condition. I make no secret that I wrote my last book because of a heartbreaking encounter I had with some former school mates who simply had no idea that reversing their type 2 diabetes and thus eliminating their need for expensive medicine was now possible. So, who can help you do that right now?

Virta Health whom we mentioned earlier is one of Rock Health's portfolio companies and they are nothing short of astonishing. As I wrote earlier, Virta Health has reversed type 2 diabetes for 60 percent of all the patients who have enrolled in their program.

Upon enrollment, Virta's members receive a box that contains a number of devices they can use to monitor their key performance indicators, including a blood glucose meter, a blood pressure cuff and a smart scale. These are connected devices that share data on members' blood sugar levels and body mass index (BMI) with a dedicated Virta care team that monitors them and remains in touch with their members. That team offers information and resources, as well as reaching out when needed to contact members when they detect that something needs to be addressed. And in reaching out, that team employs modern telehealth tools like virtual face-to-face meetings, access to 24/7 coaching, and nutrition tips to help you get and stay healthy. Their mission is reversing type 2 diabetes and they have now done so for over 50,000 customers. If any of your friends have diabetes, they absolutely need to know about companies like Virta Health.

MORE ABOUT VIRTA HEALTH

There is not only a company story but a personal story behind Virta Health. That is not unusual. In many cases, today's most innovative companies in healthcare started when their founders, or future founders, had a personal health epiphany of their own. In finding help for their ailments and diseases, those individuals embarked on personal voyages that led them to envision ways to help other people address the same health issues they were personally facing. So almost organically, a company was born. That is how Virta Health was born, when a man named Sami Inkinen confronted the reality that he was pre-diabetic.

The story of Sami and Virta Health is related on the Virta Health website. I will condense that story for you here.

In 2011, Virta's co-founder and CEO Sami Inkinen won his age group at the Ironman World Championships. But then, in that same year, he learned that he had pre-diabetes.

Sami was told the same thing that hundreds of thousands of people hear when they get the diagnosis that they are pre-diabetic, or that they have developed diabetes type 2: "Exercise more and eat less." Sami began his own studies into type 2 diabetes, which led him to Dr. Stephen Phinney and Dr. Jeff Volek, researchers into the science of carbohydrate restriction and metabolic health.

In 2014, Sami, Steve and Jeff founded Virta. To increase awareness of diabetes and pre-diabetes, Sami and his wife Meredith completed a record-breaking row from San Francisco to Hawaii.

Combining Steve and Jeff's scientific knowledge with Sami's technological expertise, Virta Health was born with an ambitious mission—to reverse type 2 diabetes in 100 million people by 2025.

In 2015, Virta launched a clinical trial in West Lafayette, Indiana, which established a "scientific foundation for type 2 diabetes reversal and Virta's unwavering commitment to being evidence-based."

Later that year, Virta publicized its first peer-reviewed manuscript, which demonstrated diabetes reversal in nearly half of the study population in as little as 10 weeks. Eighty-seven percent of patients on insulin either reduced usage or eliminated it altogether.

In 2017, Virta established an advisory board of physicians, scientists, and policy-makers. One was Dr. Don Berwick, former Administrator of the Centers for Medicare, and Medicaid Services, who joined Virta's Board of Directors.

Meanwhile, Sami and his team continued to refine the model they had developed for continuous remote care, upending traditional diabetes treatment by providing near real-time and technology-enabled access to physicians and health coaches. The Virta Treatment option expanded to every state in the nation.

By 2018, Virta's peer-reviewed results had shown diabetes reversal in 60 percent of completing patients, with 94 percent of participants reducing or eliminating insulin usage.

Due to $45 million in Series B funding, Virta doubled its team size and tripled its customer base. And in that year, Virta announced its plan to put 100 percent of their fees at risk for their enterprise partners, accelerating adoption of the Virta Treatment and bringing diabetes reversal to as many people as possible.

So what started with a personal diagnosis of pre-diabetes could well result in a major disruptive change in the way we think about treating people with diabetes.

This kind of story, while extraordinary, is actually being played out, with variations, at a growing number of young and emerging healthcare companies. What starts out as one person's personal passion can become part of history as a legendary turning point.

A few short years ago, nobody would have believed any company claiming that this could be done. Part of the credit for that accomplishment goes to the technology that Virta has applied, and to the system of monitoring and treatment which it delivers.

But part of that accomplishment can be tied to something Megan Zweig mentioned. For lack of a better term, it has happened because of a change in the way people envision what it means to have diabetes. It comes down to psychology.

Part of this change, along with the results that have followed, come from the fact that Virta Health encourages people who have type 2 diabetes to stop letting the disease define them. They don't think of themselves as "diabetics," but rather as people who have a condition that they need help with.

Companies like this have experienced a sea change. They meet people where they are. And that thinking influences the way Rock Health approaches making investments. They ask whether if what we are doing solves a real world healthcare problem and then they help companies get that into the hands of the people who need them most.

This change in thinking is a godsend. If you take a look at the core of the Rock Health mission, it means supporting innovators who are working at the intersection of healthcare and technology. They want to make healthcare massively better for everyone, driving down cost while improving services for more people.

Massively better means driving incredible change, by orders of magnitude. It's more than doing something in one dimension. They are helping us create a world where healthcare is functional, reliable, convenient, and yes, inexpensive.

Ultimately, they are forcing us to confront ourselves with tough questions like, what is expected of us? They are trying to help us build the best healthcare system in the world.

When you look at Rock Health's portfolio companies, you see a wonderful cornucopia of solutions that are tackling a lot of the problems that others have shied away from. They really dive right in and want to talk to you. They are not afraid of helping us develop solutions for people who are suffering from mental health afflictions and people who are trying to quit smoking. They do this for hospitals and health plans, employers and anyone who honestly believes they can do better population health management.

The exciting thing about Rock Health is they have an appetite for early stage investments. If you're a company that has an idea you really believe in, they will help you develop that proof of concept, get it funded, and then get it taken to market. They do so with relentless problem-solving, while providing support for you to help you grow and scale a very good idea to make it a sustainable entity. That is a huge differentiator for Rock Health.

They can help startups deal with a broad range of business and technology issues, from fundraising to go-to-market customer development, business development, contracting, pricing, business models, registering and defending intellectual property communications, and more.

It seems like everyone is trying to move an idea forward, and each player (like Rock Health) brings with them a variety of perspectives and strategic insights about healthcare that help an innovator who might be good at solving a specific problem, but not necessarily good at getting the industry to use it or even be aware of it.

What has evolved is a community of founders who can all help one another muscle through some of the tougher but common early hurdles that need to be cleared. Rock Health probably has one of the most impressive ecosystems in any industry and has become the bellwether for how to stoke innovation and launch important new ideas in healthcare. I like calling out Rock Health and giving them props, because they were first to adopt that kind of larger vision.

THE LIFELINE OF INNOVATION

We are now seeing a growing number of startup incubators that look a lot like Rock Health. Not all of them are in the San Francisco Bay Area; as we go to print, there are incubators, hot spots, and accelerators emerging throughout the United States and beyond. Israel is churning out some of the best ideas and fresh new companies anywhere. In chapter seven on life hacks, we will look at Lumen, an Israeli company that helps you tailor a diet that is best for you simply by analyzing your breath.

Kudos to Halle Tecco, founder emeritus at Rock Health and the existing team there who carry on her vision and mission. Healthcare needs more optimists. She helped create an amazing company that most think of as the straw that stirs the drink. The stories of these enablers show that if change is going to happen in healthcare, you need more than just an idea. You need funding and you need mentors. You need people who can help you identify what your intellectual property is, and what you need to do to protect it.

And you need some good old-fashioned, honest-to-goodness insight into how much money will be needed to make a vision real, into how long it is going to take, and a schedule of the achievements you will need to reach by the time you get to the end of your runway. And by the way, you need to identify a group of investors who can come in right behind your lead team, and also have an idea about who those investors and additional partners are who can help you move forward and bring your concept to market.

One of the toughest lessons we have learned is that when promising startups come to market under-funded and under-planned, they often fail. Let's face it, it takes more than solving a stubborn and persistent problem to make a real difference. It takes market acceptance and an evidence-based approach. Increasingly, consumers are finding themselves in the driver's seat of influencing our industry's direction even if it is still in subtle ways. Today's subtle can be tomorrow's left hook. If you can't help me get and stay healthy, why should you expect my business?

We have to remember that not everything in healthcare innovation is going to be a gizmo or gadget. There's a lot of heavy lifting getting done behind the scenes that makes buying healthcare solutions easy.

That is where a company like Rock Health plays a critical role in changing the landscape of American healthcare and health. We just explored how a company like Virta Health can help people with diabetes type 2 reverse their condition, thus eliminating their need for meds and unnecessary amputations. But not everything is consumer facing.

One of the fundamental pillars for how consumers can buy healthcare continues to be our state driven healthcare marketplaces or exchanges. Later, we will explore how large states like California and small states like Vermont are managing the challenge of giving consumers access to healthcare plans that meet their needs. Before we get there, let's take a look at another Rock Health portfolio company that is making all that possible.

MEET W3LL

W3LL makes the technology that drives many of our direct-to-consumer marketplaces. They are an e-commerce engine, sometimes described as the Expedia of health insurance. We caught up with Sarah Pew, General Manager and Senior Vice President of W3LL, for this section. Sarah, from Stonybrook, New York, is in many ways representative of who is pushing healthcare toward becoming a more consumer experience. At first look, her credentials don't seem to fit healthcare. She came from outside the industry, has a Fine Arts degree, spent the early part of her career as a photographer and later helped transition advertisers to digital. So how does someone who comes from an arts, manufacturing and supply chain background make the jump to healthcare? Quite nicely as it turns out. Today, Sarah will tell you what many of us in the industry already appreciate—coming from outside healthcare is exactly what healthcare needs and is probably an advantage. Show me a healthcare incumbent with consumer DNA in healthcare, I'll wait. It is difficult to disrupt from within an industry whose very idea of an ecosystem has historically begun and ended with payers and providers. Constance Sjoquist. a thought leader in the health industry, whom I interviewed for my last book *The Digital Health Revolution*, likes to say, "Healthcare needs to understand that the world is changing, and we need to change with it."

In many ways, Constance stands in the middle of this vortex, challenging incumbents to be more empathetic and sympathetic about what is missing. As an independent voice, Constance not only challenges the incumbents but the innovators as well. In a very real sense, she steps beyond strategic thinking at the 100,000-foot level and examines what's happening at the point of execution. Her challenge to companies like W3LL is simple:

How do you make the selection process simpler and easier to navigate?

Fortunately, W3LL takes that a step further, challenging itself to ask, how do we make it a delightful experience in the most compelling way possible? That is probably attributable to bringing in leadership like Sarah.

In other words, is my experience on my state's healthcare landing page similar to my experience on Amazon? It is one thing to have that as a mission, but if you are a single parent of two children, you don't care much about healthcare industry jargon. You don't really care which health plan brand to choose, you want to know the best plan that meets your family's needs. Does a plan cover mental health, drug addiction or depression? Can I strike a balance between low monthly costs and high deductibles in a way that doesn't bring me to my financial knees? To help W3LL cover those bases, Sarah tells us they like to hire people from outside the healthcare industry who can relate to what it is like being a mother, father, son, or daughter. It is refreshing to be able to have these choices served up by people who look just like us. Not everyone is from healthcare, but we all need healthcare coverage. It is little things that help us make sense of premiums, deductibles, and maximum out-of-pocket expenses.

One of my favorite thought leaders from my last book was the CEO of Wildflower Health. Leah Sparks remains one of the most inspirational leaders we have in healthcare. She is a mom first and she was frustrated by how healthcare has historically treated mothers who are the CEO of healthcare purchases in most every household. So, she started Wildflower for expecting mothers. Like all successful innovators, she has negotiated her fair share of pivots. What started as a solution for expecting mothers has morphed into a solution for family health. She takes the challenge of shopping for a plan one step further by helping parents at home find a doctor that works for them. One of the biggest challenges they have taken on is removing the baggage of an industry where your insurer defines a plan, brokers take it to market, employers purchase it, and employees select the plan. Family members are so removed from the insurer who defined the plan they have practically no say in what the plan looks like or whether it truly meets their needs.

Imagine trying to interact with a company who has historically been so far removed from you that the only time you interact is when they goof up! Companies like W3LL and Wildflower unravel that level of complexity to make it less of a convoluted process. To do that, W3LL developed a mantra that millennials can relate to: *We are mobile first.*

This company combines understanding how people shop with what drives them to your site, servicing them in a way that fully meets their needs. Is it any surprise that 70 percent of their marketplace customers arrive from their smartphones?

Wildflower develops an easy-to-navigate mobile experience and iterates based on customer feedback. Do you like how you scroll and make selections? How can we better filter information to make navigating even more easy? W3LL pays very close attention to who is using their site and how they are arriving there. This is especially important because in healthcare, that is a rarity. They also know where their customers are hanging out online, right down to their favorite social media and networking sites. This is absolutely critical for finding people where they are on the device they prefer to use.

They not only understand the diversity of their customer demographics but the differences in how different consumers expect to shop for their healthcare. As such, they have become as much a marketing partner for the marketplaces they drive as a technology partner. It is one thing for a state or maybe even AARP to provide a place to pick a plan, it is another thing entirely to understand what drives the behavior of the demographics they serve and that is what makes W3LL such a valuable part of the equation. From boomers to millennials, they get what people are looking for and how they shop. This helps anyone using W3LL to drive their marketplace to build loyalty and trust.

W3LL is quickly becoming one of the most important companies that you have never heard of. Whether you are a full-time, seasonal, or part-time employee, when logging onto your company's human resources (HR) portal, chances are, you are using a white-labeled solution driven by W3LL. W3LL helps employers integrate content via channels like YouTube to provide employees with the content they need to make informed decisions. Whether applying this concept to employers or associations like AARP, you no longer need to hunt and peck on the Internet. W3LL is aggregating suppliers and providing you with that Amazon experience we all crave in healthcare.

It should be remembered that Amazon wasn't selling everything under the sun right from the start, they started out selling books. While it is exciting to see consumer-driven marketplaces in healthcare emerge, it is even more exciting to think about how they will evolve. How cool would it be not to have to constantly provide your information to healthcare providers and everyone they partner with, every time you interact? If my health plan recommends using Noom, shouldn't Noom have a good idea of who I am when I sign-up? As we transition from sickness to wellness in healthcare, this will be huge.

CHAPTER THREE

MEET THE NEW DISRUPTORS

It is fun checking in on the companies who are delivering healthcare services and solutions to consumers and meeting them where they are. Some of those end-users are using apps on their phones. Others are opening boxes from their healthcare providers and unpacking smart scales, smart glucose monitors, and other devices that connect them directly to remote coaches and caregivers who can monitor them and help keep them healthy.

No doubt about it, many of those services are being delivered right to your door as a bundle. It is easy to imagine a world where everything in healthcare is connected to enable high levels of care. As COVID is proving, sometimes that means without ever physically interacting directly with other people.

But for all our technological advancement in connectivity, another trend that is evolving has more to do with real-life settings and daily interactions. This includes retail pharmacies, walk-in health clinics, nutritionists' offices, and weight-loss specialists, as well as food stores.

THE MERGER OF TECHNOLOGY AND PERSONAL EXPERIENCES

Digital may be the new front door, but face-to-face care is not going away. Digital health is extending how we can monitor progress and manage interventions, but in-person care can be found right in your local neighborhood. You would expect COVID to lead to a feeling of isolation, yet innovative retailers and care providers are making getting care as easy as going to the market for groceries.

How retail pharmacy uses digital health is probably one of the most fascinating developments in healthcare. Our local stores have figured out how to create a longitudinal relationship with us that is influenced by their first-hand view of our health data over time. From devices to analytics, to health management, diagnostics, and testing, the result is a new range of care choices you can access in person from your laptop, on your phone and in your neighborhood. In many cases, no appointment is necessary, walk-ins are welcomed. For a mom pressed for time who is out shopping with her children, being able to pop in for vaccinations just because you are in the neighborhood is huge. As retailers expand their physical and digital offerings, you get a sense that they are becoming the local hub for you to access care, monitor results and get help when you need it. Having the store local means having a local provider who knows you. Staying connected via digital tools you use from your phone opens up a whole new world of care possibilities.

Who are the disruptors driving the retail trend?

MEET TORBEN NIELSEN,
CHIEF EXECUTIVE OFFICER, ZOOMCARE

Torben Nielsen is a true visionary in the world of distributed healthcare. He is the CEO of ZoomCare, one of the most innovative and exciting new companies that there is. It has expanded steadily since it opened its first walk-in clinic in Tigard, Oregon, in 2006. There are now more than 60 clinics in Oregon and Washington, with plans to add more and expand into neighboring states. And over the years, ZoomCare has added a unique and user-friendly telehealth platform to its neighborhood clinics. ZoomCare has quickly become part of the local community.

"Our clinics are what make us unique in the world of healthcare," says Torben, who joined ZoomCare in 2019. And he is right, because ZoomCare's blend of telehealth and physical clinics is powerful.

ZoomCare offers instant telehealth services on phones, computers, and tablets. And instant means *instant*, because members can have telehealth consultations with ZoomCare physicians in a matter of seconds. And if a member needs to see a physician face-to-face in a clinic, that happens not only same day if needed, but usually as soon as the member can get to a ZoomCare clinic. That helps explain why ZoomCare was voted "Best Primary Doctor" in *Willamette Week's* 2017 readers' poll.

BRINGING THE 21ST CENTURY
TO CONSUMERS OF HEALTHCARE SERVICES

"As you can tell from my accent," Torben tells us, "I wasn't born and raised in the U.S. I'm a good Danish-speaking boy and I'm going to date myself by saying that I came to the U.S. years ago as an exchange student. I fell in love with a girl from California and the rest of it is history. Now my wife and I have three girls.

"I have a favorite saying about healthcare: I work in healthcare during the day and then I go home to the 21st century.

"Let's think about that. The fact is, healthcare for the most part has been stuck back in the 20th century. But in our homes and many other aspects of our lives, we are well into the 21st century. And our patients or consumers have been yearning for, and asking us for, much more of the kind of 21st century experience they have when they are using Amazon.com, eBay, Yelp or any one of many 21st century offerings."

Torben explains that although healthcare consumers want to have access to information, they also want to enjoy an experience that's real. That can be achieved, he believes, when companies use technology in the right way.

"These days," Torben says, "who goes on the web using a computer? We now do it by using our phones. And that is where ZoomCare is now. It's a 15-year-old company, but it was built from the ground up with technology in mind. And I think that is what is setting us up for a really strong connection to our consumers."

MEET SARAH

Torben and his team at ZoomCare have created an archetype who represents the company's patient. Torben and his team call her "Sarah." In meetings, the ZoomCare team members talk about her, have meetings about her, and feel that they know her. Sarah personifies the customer that ZoomCare Is serving.

And Sarah has become so real that everyone on Torben's team really "knows" her. Sarah is a busy mom. She has kids. She has a household where she is the "CEO of healthcare," the person in charge. But Sarah, as envisioned by Torben and his team, is also a working professional.

And how does Sarah want her healthcare?

- She wants it *where* she wants it, *when* she wants it.

- She wants it to be delivered by a *professional*.

- She wants to know what the *price point* is.

"That's similar to what consumers want when dealing with companies in any other modern industry," Torben tells us.

And that's what ZoomCare is striving to deliver—an experience that allows a consumer like Sarah to get her healthcare taken care of, where she wants it, when she wants it. And in a very seamless manner.

And the interesting thing is that Sarah can't anticipate when she's going to want or need healthcare. When one of her children needs care, she wants it right then.

Torben explains, "That's the difference between healthcare and, say, travel. I mean, if I am booking travel, I can start looking at my options 30 days in advance. I can shop to get the best price. I've got time to research it. But if my child's sick, I wasn't planning for that to happen. And boom, it does, and then my needs are immediate. Sure, some of our in-clinic appointments are scheduled ahead of time. But 85 percent of the in-clinic appointments we schedule take place within four hours. That's what Sarah needs, and we orient our company around that."

TORBEN REFLECTS ON SARAH'S NEIGHBORHOOD

"Our system is built around your neighborhood," Torben tells us. "We now have 60 clinics in neighborhoods in Portland and Seattle, and in between. And we have a physical footprint in small little neighborhood clinics.

"And do you know what? Many consumers are discovering that they can have their kids taken care of at home, via telehealth. We've seen tremendous growth, a tremendous uptick. It's not asynchronous where you log in and leave a message that says, 'Hey, my kid has a rash. Can somebody get back to me, maybe tomorrow?'

"No, in maybe 10 or 15 seconds you can see someone on chat, who can look at your kid's rash. You get access to a provider right away. And we have found that in certain cases, it is better to embed a photo so a provider can look at it, enlarge it if need be. That works better than a video.

"It's like a suitcase. We provide primary care. We provide urgent care. And we provide specialty care.

"We develop most of our software ourselves. We have a really sophisticated development team, and we are investing heavily in it so we can create a seamless experience, one that's connected, from virtual to the clinics to our EMR to the personal timeline or personal health record that sits in an app.

"And we have our own pharmacy. We can prescribe medicines and have them delivered to your home. Soon, we will be able to do that same day. And it's all connected and tied into the app. We will know when you need a refill. We know how you're doing on the meds. And it's a seamless, connected system.

"We have found that developing technology in-house is the way to go. It's how we best provide a seamless and up-to-date experience.

"There is a heavy software component to what we do. We're developing technologies to differentiate our provider capabilities, as opposed to wanting to be a tech firm that sells or licenses its technologies to other companies."

THE GROWTH OF
TELEMEDICINE DURING THE PANDEMIC

"We're seeing tremendous traction on telehealth as an industry, which is really great," Torben continues.

"For a little history, long before the pandemic, we launched phone care. It took off right away. And then we launched video, and the same thing happened. And now we're doing telehealth and over the past four months, we have done 40,000 telehealth visits, which is incredible for us as a regional player.

"And telehealth is continuing to change. Currently, 34 percent of our telehealth visits actually come from outside the areas where we have clinics, which is phenomenal. All of a sudden, we are seeing new people pop up in our telehealth channels. And they love it. Telehealth is beginning to feel more like a workflow automation tool and not necessarily a 'pick up your phone and call somebody' kind.

"If I can elaborate on that, we think of it as an integral part of that seamless consumer experience. We know that about 20 percent of care actually cannot be provided in a telehealth solution. You may need imaging at some point, or you may need labs. Or you may need to have a doctor actually look at you. That can't be done in telehealth. We think that part of our advantage is that we can take what's happening in a telehealth setting and we can schedule a same-day appointment for you at a neighborhood clinic.

"The clinic could be right across the street from where you're having your telehealth chat, and you just walk in. And it's a seamless, integrated experience. And then, for our archetype Sarah, the data and the records for that visit are all going to be sitting on her personal health record as part of the app.

"Sarah doesn't even need to think about her password, because these days, our users are using face ID technology. Easy, immediate access is built into the whole process. Boise, Denver, and Boulder will be three new markets for us. The Denver, Colorado, market is similar to what our Seattle markets are. And we felt that that would be a good expansion."

BUILDING RELATIONSHIPS WITH CONSUMERS

"We have 100 percent app adoption, which is incredible," Torben explains. "That means that all of our members utilize our app on their phones, or they log in on the web. That means we have a relationship with them.

"Even when we have people walking into our clinics off the street, we try to build relationships with them. If they don't have our app or they haven't set up a profile yet, we help them do that if they want to. They will get set up in the system, so they have an account and a profile. And that allows us to have communication with them and to build a relationship over time.

"We can remind them of medication refills, for instance. We can remind them that they haven't had their annual physical or that it is time for a flu shot. And we're starting to look at more sophisticated data analysis to identify care that should be delivered. We are moving into that space, and we think that there will be big benefits. I think being able to move quickly to accurately analyze information is probably right at the top of the list of priorities, right? We'll get that built, based on AI and machine learning. It just feels like further automation of healthcare."

TOWARD CONTEXTUAL HEALTHCARE

"If you have somebody on video on their phone," says Torben, "you can ask them, 'What does your fridge look like right now . . . .can you show me?'

"You can ask people to show you the food they have in their fridges or show you the medicines they're taking. And that provides context for the overall care that we couldn't do when people walk into the clinic. And that allows us to provide better care."

ATTACKING CARE DISCREPANCIES

"I think absolutely there's an opportunity for us in some of the neighborhoods and populations that have been overlooked. And we've talked a lot about that, especially with regard to Black Lives Matter," Torben says.

"We are focusing on health disparities now. Are there communities where we should be a much more active player? Yes, we want ZoomCare to be a driving neighborhood advocate, taking action into how to best manage health disparities in that particular neighborhood. Telehealth, coupled with clinics, could let us do that. And what do we need to do to really go after that, to serve those communities? That is a question we are thinking about every day."

A VISIT TO THE NEW CVS

If you live just about anywhere in the continental United States, you can probably walk from your home to a CVS store. And if you've been a CVS customer for more than a year or two, you have already noticed very big changes taking place. A few years ago, you might have noticed that you could get a flu shot right in your CVS pharmacy. And chances are that may have surprised you. You might have also noticed that your store had opened a walk-in clinic where you could ask questions, receive a range of care, and enjoy the ability to postpone going to your primary care-providing physician.

Those changes, which were so new only a few years ago, are no longer surprising. They have become part of what we have come to expect from our local CVS pharmacies. Let's hear from former CVS executive Justin Steinman.

In many ways, Justin is exactly what healthcare needs. He challenges norms and has a curiosity driven nature. He doesn't just look at a particular situation and diagnose the problem. He is already game-planning the top three ways to solve it. In short, he is exactly who you want at the helm when defining and managing new complex initiatives that are expected to scale. Justin started his healthcare career at GE Medical and then transitioned to Aetna just prior to their merger with CVS. Back then, not many saw health plans and retail pharmacy merging on their bingo card. Their customer value proposition changed overnight. The mother of all integrations was on, and Justin was right in the thick of it.

HOW "BRICKS AND CLICKS" COMBINE TO CREATE A UNIFIED CUSTOMER CARE EXPERIENCE

Vertical integration was one of the key issues that CVS addressed. CVS was essentially in the retail business. There were so many CVS stores and at a certain point, management realized that selling magazines and greeting cards did not support a long-term growth strategy.

It was at that point that a new kind of thinking arose, when CVS decided to reposition itself not as a retailer, but as "the front door to healthcare in America," Justin explains.

And another kind of integration was taking place too, around the issue of payments.

"If you're going to spend that dollar on preventative care in the store," Justin says, "but you're going to save $1.50 on the insurance medical costs, it makes a lot of sense to do the deal."

Among the first integration products CVS launched were the MinuteClinics that opened in CVS locations across the country. The planning for them was backed up with market research that showed that a lot of CVS customers were people who were making less than $50,000 a year. And for those people, the cost of care was proving to be a significant inhibitor to getting care. The strategy behind the MinuteClinics was to offer a care option that costs about $100 to consumers—far less than the cost of at least $200 to them at an emergency room. The value and convenience would speak to consumers. And the proposition was just as appealing to employers and the health plans they used, considering the cost for every visit to an emergency room is at least $4,000.

Justin explains, "So we had an idea. You could walk into a MinuteClinic, show them your Aetna card, and there would be no cost to you for that visit at all. Your employer is going to pay for it, at absolutely no out-of-pocket cost to you. Justin and his planning team modeled that would save an employer something on the order of about 13 cents per member per month. So Aetna added this feature to its program, which covered about four million members. If you do the math, you can see the savings and the value.

FROM PHYSICAL TO VIRTUAL AND BACK AGAIN

The Aetna/CVS cooperation has resulted in a vision of unified care. "We at CVS liked to say only CVS has the ability to go from virtual to physical to virtual and back again," says Justin. "We talked a lot about the omni-channel approach to meeting members where they are. Another product that we built is now called Virtual Primary Care. And this is a new plan design that we built."

Part of the thinking was to overcome consumer objections to telemedicine. The greatest of those objections, Justin states, is that consumers feel they never see the same doctor twice. "And people who say that are right," he says. "To date, telemedicine has been episodic. You sprain your ankle, you use Teledoc and you see someone online. Same with a sore throat. Only every time you call, you see someone else! Maybe the doctors you see are actually moonlighters, or they might not be the people who file your paperwork. And maybe your company is paying for it, but there are a million reasons why you're not going to like it."

One solution the CVS/Aetna team developed was to move data from the primary care practice to the cloud—not only data from the primary care doctor, but from nurse practitioners as well—so everyone can access it.

A REALITY-BASED WAY
TO RESEARCH NEEDED CHANGES

The Aetna/CVS team took notebooks and visited their primary care providers. They tracked what needed to be done physically and made notes about what could be done virtually at a wellness telemedicine visit.

"In truth, there are certain things at a wellness visit that you need done physically, face to face," Justin explains. "You have your reflexes checked. The caregiver feels your lymph nodes to see if they are normal. Or someone takes your blood. But our experiments showed that roughly 85 percent of what happens can be done virtually, including the entire conversation with the primary care physician." And they concluded that all but 15 percent of those care experiences could be performed via telemedicine, and even more at MediClinics like those that CVS was planning to install in stores.

Before COVID-19, CVS was on track to build 1,000 of those health hubs around the country. And now, post-COVID-19, CVS is planning to install about 5,000 by the year 2025. So now all of a sudden, the customer gets a better care experience. And employers or insurance providers will save money and keep people healthier too.

It really goes from physical to virtual, and back again. It is seamlessly omni-channel, all working because there is a vertically integrated set of assets.

AETNA ADVICE: ONE MORE WAY AETNA
AND CVS WILL STAY A STEP AHEAD
OF END-USERS' CARE NEEDS

Aetna Advice is a series of algorithms that uses data analytics to determine the next best action for customers' health. In this way,

CVS hopes to become a leading center for early interventions for diabetes and other conditions.

And the whole system will be automated. If users have Apple Watches, for example, they will receive reminders and alerts there. Of course, text messaging and email will be part of the communications.

When CVS customers are in the store and picking up prescriptions, the plan is for them to receive messages that might say, "You haven't had a flu shot for two years. Why not go get one right now?" Timely and on point, they nudge you to do the preventative at a time when it is most convenient.

Another real life example is when your physician prescribes an MRI, that information will enter the CVS system and consumers will get a text message that says, "Would you like to get an MRI at a center that's nearby? It's covered, and it will cost you $500, vs. $3,000 at your local hospital. Click here and schedule it right now?"

ON CVS'S CURRENT INVOLVEMENT IN COVID-19 TESTING

CVS is currently cooperating with a number of businesses to perform COVID-19 tests on their employees. One such partner is a major airline, which is having pilots tested at some of their major hubs. There is also a contract with a major television studio, which is testing production people, actors, and even catering workers.

According to Justin, one of the major stock exchanges is another client. It is giving Covid-19 screening tests to traders on the floor, to maintenance people in their facilities—to everyone on site. Another partner is a medical device company that sends reps into operating rooms.

What's the common thread across those segments? It is how densely people work together. It's a vertical integration, not a typical segmentation.

It is all evolving into a white-glove service that combines the resources of CVS and Aetna.

NOW, LET'S SEE WHAT WALGREENS IS DOING

Lately, Walgreens has come to be known as the Walgreens Boots Alliance, or WBA.

If you live in most parts of America, you might think that CVS and Walgreens pharmacy stores are similar. They are all conveniently located, probably only a short drive from your home. They are surrounded by adequate parking and often equipped with drive-through windows where you can drop off and pick up prescriptions. And when you walk inside, you find a modern, spacious, and well-lit space where you can shop for cosmetics, health supplies, and even a range of goods that were sold principally in groceries, until recently. And of course, there is a pharmacy counter.

If you live or travel to other countries, however, you realize that Walgreens is global. In fact, Walgreens currently has more than 2,300 stores in the UK, more than 1,100 stores in Mexico, as well as stores in Chile, Thailand, Norway, the Netherlands, and even Lithuania.

So, one difference is that Walgreens is more of an international concern and therefore can harvest lessons learned in healthcare using global data points. But that is not the only difference, as we learn from Giovanni Monti, Senior Vice President, Healthcare Services for Walgreens Boots Alliance. When we interviewed Giovanni, he was in Italy where he lives and works. Walgreens has more than just stores throughout the world. Their leadership team represents their international flair as well.

"As the SVP for Healthcare Services at WBA," Giovanni says, "I lead a business connecting individuals to healthcare solutions and services, providers, and payers, online and in their community. With teams in Chicago and Deerfield, Seattle, London and

Nottingham, WBA Healthcare Services offers healthcare solutions via Walgreens Find Care, the care navigation and management digital platform, via neighborhood healthcare destinations that we are developing across Walgreens, and at Boots in the UK and in Europe.

"Solutions comprise primary care partnerships, including VillageMD, LabCorp, weight management solutions from Jenny Craig, digital therapeutics and connected care products, pharmacogenomics and a number of other health services.

"Prior to leading WBA Healthcare Services, I co-founded the WBA Healthcare Innovation Platform, that I continue to lead, which has developed healthcare innovations across the U.S. and Europe. I joined WBA as Director of Corporate Development and Mergers & Acquisitions (M&A) in 2012, with previous experience in corporate development, M&A, and management consulting.

"I started pushing for a few different healthcare solutions, whether it was point-of-care technology or genomics or new tech-enabled healthcare services. And I guess the company liked it, because after a while I created what is called the Healthcare Platform—a global team that I still run. After a while, we started to build a healthcare marketplace in the U.S. I was really focusing back then on digital healthcare in the U.S.

"At some point, the company decided to bring together healthcare and digital, which is when they asked me to lead healthcare services, including all the partnerships that we have with VillageMD and a number of other partners."

HOW WBA USES DATA

Giovanni and his team are doing more and more to develop a better view of customers and serve them better. Among his team's innovations are something called a Health Outcomes Pharmacist.

This program plays a special role, managing people whose data earmarks them as being more at risk than other Walgreens customers.

Based on that data, a determination is made about whether there is anything that Walgreens needs to do in a number of areas, including medications, arrangements with payers, and more. "That's all data-driven," Giovanni explains. "And it relies on the ability not just to read and analyze data, but to share it across the various partners of the healthcare continuum."

And innovative thinking continues to evolve. For example, WBA has just announced an agreement with Adobe. The goal is to help Walgreens develop an even more precise, personalized, and inclusive view of customers, that will bring together data from every interaction with them." Across immunization . . . everything," Giovanni says, "with the goal of developing a more personalized engagement with customers."

VILLAGE MEDICAL AND THE CHANGING ROLE OF THE PRIMARY CARE PROVIDER

To make Walgreens stores personalized and impactful on health outcomes, Giovanni and his team have decided that the primary care provider is the place to start.

They have decided that primary care providers can have the biggest impact on the lives of healthcare consumers. And something else, too. Primary care providers can also have the greatest impact on all the other entities that operate within the healthcare ecosystem. They work with patients, with pharmacies, with healthcare plans, and with everyone else.

That explains why Walgreens has recently made a big investment in VillageMD, with a goal of soon having between 500 and 700 co-located Village Medical clinics installed in Walgreens stores.

"Village is where we'll develop that integration between

primary care and pharmacy," Giovanni explains. "And it is not just a physical co-location, but an integration across all the channels that we have available. Because the care we are delivering—and we want to deliver more and more, again with VillageMD—is where it makes sense for individuals. It can be through our app, at home, in the co-located practices. We're excited. We have just announced it, and it also fits very well with the title of your book."

WALGREENS FIND CARE

Walgreens has also launched a new app called Walgreens Find Care. In concept, it is more than just an app—it is a digital healthcare marketplace that end users carry around with them on their phones.

Giovanni and his development team see it as the digital, interactive front door to healthcare where customers will find care based on who they are and the solutions they find will be from Walgreens and its partners. A broad selection of care will reside in the app, including general telehealth, acute care, specialist care, continuous glucose monitoring, and more.

"Regardless of whether we or our partners provide the solutions," Giovanni says, "and regardless of whether online or through physical services or a lab, it's all driven by that personal understanding of the individual and what makes sense for him or her, based on their healthcare needs at that time. We believe that combining a personal digital front end with the most relevant personal healthcare interaction with the primary care physician (PCP) can be a powerful way to increase access to healthcare through the most efficient channel, based on the specific need. And again, with the goal of ultimately improving outcome and reducing cost. In fact, we are focused on net promoter scores. We want an experience that is as pleasant as possible."

READINESS AND RESPONSIVENESS TO COVID-19

"The investment we have made in building digital assets and the digital front door has been tremendously helpful over the last few months," Giovanni says. "No one ever expected something like Covid-19. But thanks to how ready we were, in a matter of days we very significantly increased the offering of telehealth solutions. We launched a Covid-19 risk assessment tool, based on Microsoft. In a matter of days, we delivered COVID-19 drive-through tests because we had built the digital front end to reach the Walgreens customer.

"We're making sure that we're able to distribute all the equipment that's necessary and needed in each country and jurisdiction, that we do all the testing that is required and possible. We are creating the necessary awareness and of course, we have done a huge amount just to keep pharmacies open every day in every community in the dozens of countries where we operate. A huge effort, but it's been very much appreciated by our customers and everyone we deal with.

"Because of the pandemic, it is fascinating to see how healthcare has changed in just the last few months. It is going to change even more in the coming years, but it is already totally different. You have read about how many years healthcare has accelerated in just a few months. But we can see that awareness in the adoption of digital health solutions, and people's willingness to interact with doctors online if desired, if needed. I think we have 14 times the number of users we had and not even in our most ambitious plans would we have expected that. And it's not only that. It's also the adoption of AI-powered solutions, it's the adoption of what we just discussed earlier. The power of a point-of-care diagnostic. And how it's been quickly deployed across different delivery channels, including Walgreens drive-throughs."

It goes to show that the kind of digital solutions that Walgreens has developed will also help the company to adapt to any healthcare crises and needs that may arrive in the future.

THE CHANGING FACE OF DIGITAL HEALTHCARE

Giovanni sums up Walgreens' presence in the digital landscape:

"We started engaging people in a . . . I don't want to say a *modern* way, that's wrong. But in healthcare, like what has happened in travel and so many industries, people are expecting to interact using their smart phones. This will make technology even more important. And our partnership with Microsoft is enabling us to do so much more, and much more quickly. We are leveraging digital health technologies to make healthcare much more personal. It's not just a doctor who is sitting in front of a computer. You really have your own interaction, powered by technology.

"In our Find Care app, there is a very rich partner and care roadmap. I think that roadmap, powered by technology, is becoming more personalized and predictive. Because the more we know about individuals, the more data-driven care becomes, the more relevant we can be in managing populations and partnering with a variety of players that bear the cost of management."

KEY ALLIANCES THAT BENEFIT THE CONSUMER

Walgreens currently has nutritionists available in about 100 locations, with plans to expand well beyond that. And if that weren't enough, Jenny Craig nutrition and weight loss counselors are on-site too.

In addition, Walgreens has forged an alliance with Kroger, a leading American food store chain.

Think of this as a unified, integrated, flowing kind of customer experience.

Let's say that a man visits a VillageMD clinic, complaining of fatigue. His name is Paul. An attending physician there recommends tests, which determine that Paul has pre-diabetes. So, in addition to getting a prescription for Metformin (an oral medication that is commonly prescribed for pre-diabetes and type 2 diabetes), Paul also visits a nutritionist with Jenny Craig at VillageMD. Together, Paul and the counselor work out a plan for a healthy week's worth of meals. Paul then goes to the Kroger store located adjacent to the pharmacy, where a Kroger's shopper already has a basket of foods that the Jenny Craig counselor forwarded to her. Paul has successfully navigated another week of eating healthfully. It is easy to imagine meals being delivered right to Paul's door. Meals prescribed by VillageMD, delivered by Krogers and nutrition tips, tricks and traps provided by Jenny Craig. The "corner of happy and healthy" has done it again!

It's unified, personal, yet supported by a range of technological tools.

Only a few years ago, this kind of experience would not have been possible. Today, it is becoming the new normal. Walgreens is using data from all their interactions to better help you live the healthiest life possible. They make the marriage of bricks and clicks work from a very practical and measurable perspective. While Find Care is Walgreen's digital front door, what it connects you to has depth and breadth. It is here where you see their joint ventures, investments and organic solutions shine. Understanding how to influence and sustain behavior change using real world data is like having a super power in healthcare. Sometimes, the tools Walgreens uses to help us aren't even things we need to download or register to use.

CATCHING UP WITH VIM

About two years ago while writing my first book, I interviewed Oron Afek, co-founder and CEO of Vim. Since then, Vim has certainly not stood still in moving forward with expanded services and agreements in the marketplace.

Yet not everything has changed. To be specific, Vim has not departed from its vision, which remains intact. As Oron explains it, when we spoke back then, Vim is a company that partners with medical providers and health systems to provide convenience, cost savings and a better care experience for patients.

"Back then, we were really just getting started," Oron tells me. But how have they pivoted and evolved?

"The goal remains getting patients to high-value care," Oron says. "That means guiding and moving episodes of care to high-performing physicians that will perform at lower costs and achieve better outcomes. That vision still remains."

Vim's goal has expanded. One new area of focus is what Oron calls "educating" consumers of healthcare and influencing their behavior. Oron stresses that getting consumers to change their patterns of behavior is challenging.

Nutrition is an evolving example. In Oron's words, "Food is medicine."

There are a lot of companies that are trying to help us get and stay healthy using food and nutrition as a foundational pillar. Walgreens, through partnerships with Kroger, Jenny Craig, VillageMD and now Vim is a great example.

Walgreens is using an ecosystem approach combining the value add-ons of coaching, digital and physical, to help their customers. VillageMD allows them to focus on getting physicians to influence their patients' behaviors and actually prescribe foods specifically designed for people with cardiometabolic conditions. Vim's focus was already on the consumer/physician relationship and was a natural fit. Why not start from that position of strength when striving to influence people's choice of foods?

"How do we optimize decisions made by doctors, caregivers and those who influence the patients?" Oron asks. "How can we influence and guide them? We realized that in order to do so, we needed to share data with physicians, but we also needed to make it into a workflow."

Oron believes that building on those three factors—workflow, multi-payer, and making our health data actionable—will help Vim achieve its goals of guiding us to a better care experience, and ultimately, better outcomes.

"Workflow is really hard from a technical perspective," according to Oron. "I mean, typically, the systems providers are using are outdated. They are really hard to integrate in a meaningful way that would help make our health data actionable. And then multi-payer is another aspect that nobody has been able to figure out, because you need to sign contracts with all the large players. You can then focus on provider engagement and say, 'Hey, I can deliver data to recommend next best action at the point of care.'"

GETTING TO SCALE

Oron and Vim made what he calls a "big pivot" toward retail health in this last year.

"We said, 'Let's build a platform and integrate with 2,000 or 3,000 physicians,'" he explains. And there are around five million clinical users in the U.S., who make clinical decisions. You might say, there are only about 1.2 million physicians. But what about nurses? There are so many other people who make clinical recommendations. Enter the pharmacist.

"We estimated that we were going to serve about five million users, and we asked, how will we ever be able to integrate with those five million? Given the fact that it takes between 12 and 18 months to finalize agreements with EMR (Electronic Medical Records) vendors, how would we ever finalize agreements with five million of them?"

Vim is now developing new technologies that allow them to integrate needed changes in a much more rapid fashion, by leveraging a number of advanced technologies.

"If we can get those 18 months of integration time down to, say, 90 seconds—and we believe we can do that—we will achieve scale in record time. So overall, despite the challenges, I would say that I am optimistic, and our prospects are very good."

KEY ALLIANCES

The Vim team are forging a number of alliances with other companies across a broad spectrum that includes retailers, insurers, care providers, and more. When they first started out, adding these other healthcare incumbents wasn't so obvious, but given that roughly 75 percent of the U.S. population lives within five miles of a Walgreens store, connecting to retail health was probably inevitable.

Here is a story line that provides a glimpse of the kind of end-user experience that will result:

"Let's think about a chronically ill patient who sees her primary care provider three times a year on average," Oron says. "But that same patient will see a pharmacist 13 times a year on average. And she might visit a convenience store a couple of times a week. But in sum, about 13 out of an average of those 23 retail experiences a year take place with a pharmacist.

"If you could generate the pharmacist type of engagement with a digital app, you could solve huge problems. But people don't use their healthcare applications too often."

Oron also cites the fact that consumers often place a lot of trust in what their pharmacists recommend. In fact, end-users sometimes trust pharmacists more than they trust their primary care providers. Plus, that pharmacist will probably know some important things about your health, like when you had your last flu shot, when you had your last colonoscopy or mammogram, your last Pap smear. In many cases, this is information that even a healthcare insurance plan will not be able to provide. Pharmacies are destined to continue to serve as really important touchpoints in the future of healthcare.

"We want to do one thing and do it really, really well," Oron says. "And that one thing is to make sure that people go to the right places to monitor and maintain good health." By the looks of things, Vim is achieving those goals. Two years after releasing *The Digital Health Revolution*, Vim remains one of the most promising and exciting companies in healthcare that you have never heard of. Maybe that is how it should be. The road to better health outcomes is getting less bumpy. There will always be room in healthcare for companies who help reduce the friction of consuming and servicing our needs.

CHAPTER FOUR
RETHINKING NUTRITION

"Let food be your medicine . . .
and your medicine be your food."
—Hippocrates, who lived from about 460-375 BCE

"Dis-moi ce que tu manges, je te dirai ce que tu es." ("Tell me
what you eat, and I will tell you what you are.")
—Anthelme Brillat-Savarin, French scientist, writing in 1826

"Der Mensch ist, was er isst." ("A man is what he eats.")
-Ludwig Andreas Feuerbach, German scientist, writing in 1864

"You Are What You Eat."
—Title of a book by the American nutritionist
Victor Lindlahr, 1942

As these quotes show, the idea that people are made up of what they eat has been around for quite a while.

That is true in a chemical sense. If you consume arsenic or mercury, it will build up in your cells and poison or kill you. If you eat too many fats, you will build up fatty tissue. If you eat too much red meat, your heart (which is made up of meaty muscle) could become unhealthy. And on it goes. The substances you eat don't pass through your system without leaving something behind. Something they contain stays on inside of you, often in unhealthy ways. They actually become part of your body.

But there is more to it than that. The expression "you are what you eat" has come to mean something slightly different today:

"Your health is determined by what you eat."

This concept has become so widely accepted, it is hard to think that as recently as half a century ago, most people were pretty unaware of the intimate connection between diet and health. To see how that concept was once outside the mainstream, consider the revolutionary effect that a nutritionist named Adelle Davis (1904-1974) had when she wrote books like *Vitality Through Planned Nutrition* (1942), *Let's Cook It Right* (1947), *Let's Eat Right to Keep Fit* (1954), *Let's Stay Healthy: A Guide to Lifelong Nutrition* (1981) and her other books.

Today, the concepts of those books have become completely mainstream. It is now hard to imagine how controversial they seemed when they were published. Davis was dismissed as a "health food nut," and even accused of being somewhat un-American when her book *Vitality Through Planned Nutrition* was published in 1942, a time when young American soldiers were heading off to war. Who was Adelle Davis to write that the red meat, mashed potatoes, and butter-soaked string beans their mothers were serving them were unhealthy? We had fighting to do, not steaming vegetables.

Well, let's fast forward to the last few decades, to today, a time when we hear over and over about the good and bad ways we are selecting and preparing our foods. Sometimes, conflicting information seems to arrive, barrage-style. Just when it becomes part of popular wisdom that eggs, butter, and whole milk will clog our arteries and inflate our cholesterol, we hear that just the opposite is true. Just when we accept the idea that alcoholic beverages will send us to an early grave, experts tell us that a glass of red wine every day is good for us.

Perhaps one of the drivers of the new, widespread zeal to understand diet and nutrition is the fact that in the last few decades, Americans are becoming increasingly overweight, and clinically obese in epidemic numbers. Even if broad swaths of the population aren't thinking about eating healthy foods, they are worried about dieting to lose weight.

Even if people doubt all the latest nutritional advice from "health nuts," they seem to accept the obvious fact that one way to lose weight is to eat less, or to eat certain foods instead of others. Yes, they want to be thinner. Yes, they want to look attractive and healthy. And if the way to achieve those goals is to think about nutrition—or accept advice and counseling about nutrition— then they will accept the idea that like it or not, it's time to think about what they eat.

ENTER COMMERCIAL DIETING ASSISTANCE AND FOODS

It's no secret that as soon as profit-centered commercial enterprises discover a widespread demand, they rush in to develop products and services to meet it. It should come as no surprise that in the 1950s—not long after Adelle Davis promulgated the idea that if people ate certain foods and beverages and avoided others, they would lose weight and be healthier and more attractive—a wide variety of new diet foods started to hit supermarket shelves.

Sugar-free sodas like Tab, which had been marketed to people with diabetes previously, were suddenly repositioned as "diet" beverages that would help people lose weight. Soon, supermarket shelves began to fill with sugar-free alternatives. Skim milk appeared. And weight-loss products arrived too. In about 1950, a company started to market a weight-loss mint called Ayds. Mead Johnson started selling a milky diet beverage called Metrical.

It was off to the races, with large numbers of people discovering the value of healthy food and the role that eating well could play in losing weight. A new kind of enterprise—the health food store—appeared on Main Streets across the country. And suddenly "fad diets," which actually began in appearance-obsessed meccas like Hollywood, started to gain adherents. Starting in the

1920s, people could choose from fads that included a grapefruit diet, a lemonade diet, and even a cigarette diet.

But those aberrant crazes were about to move toward the mainstream because people were finding that eating the right foods did more than help them shed pounds. Eating right also helped them control chronic conditions like diabetes, prevent the onset of disease, and even live longer and more energetically.

Now that principle has moved to the center of our national way of thinking about health and healthcare. It seems that everyone who wants to be healthy thinks about what they are eating today—and what a wonderful thing that is.

And in our time of digital healthcare, all kinds of innovative enterprises are moving in to help people make healthy decisions about what they eat. Healthcare providers, pharmacies, hospitals, and health insurance plans have all started to cooperate and forge commercial agreements with one another. No doubt, nutrition and diet have moved from the edges of society to the epicenter. Let's meet some of the innovators who have driven that change, and who will continue to do so in the coming years.

MEET DAVID PASTRANA, CEO, JENNY CRAIG

David Pastrana comes naturally to his career with Jenny Craig. He was born and grew up in Madrid, where he and his community practiced what he calls a Mediterranean diet that centered on eating fish, complex carbohydrates, and foods prepared with healthy olive oil.

David studied engineering and started his business career with Zara, a women's fashion brand and retailer, where he worked on marketing strategy for a number of years. What is the connection between women's fashion and weight control?

"Women's fashion is what I call an emotional women's business," David explains, "meaning that the goal is to help women feel good about themselves."

And David, like other executives we talk with in this book, had a personal epiphany about his own health. "I went through a personal health and weight loss journey myself," he says. "It was a point in my life when I had to lose about 30 pounds. I used to do a lot of sports since I was a child, and there was a point in time when I got to be close to 200 pounds. My second child had been born. I already had one who was three years old, and I realized that I couldn't continue that way. I couldn't do any sports! I had essentially focused everything on my career. I was a president of a multi-billion-dollar business, but I didn't have any time for my wife or my kids. And essentially, I didn't have any time for me."

David began what he calls "a personal weight-loss journey."

"The first thing that I stopped was coffee, and coffee became something of a learning point for me. You have a coffee in the morning, you have one in the middle of the morning, and you have one in the afternoon, and you basically get completely addicted to it. I felt like I had to get that under control. I then eliminated a lot of carbohydrates. I went back to the diet that I had eaten when I was a child and I got into exercise. I do cross training now, and I've done competitive exercise. I wanted to take the weight off for my family to be a good dad, to give to my kids and to be a good leader. When you are a president of an organization, you are managing thousands of people. You have to be extremely upbeat. You have to be happy. You have to have enjoyable conversations. You have to sleep properly. And amazingly in parallel, Jenny Craig was an opportunity that became available to me. I was extremely excited because it's essentially the journey that I'll be working on for the rest of my life."

DISCOVERING PREVENTIVE MEDICINE AND CARE

David conceptualizes weight loss as a branch of preventive medicine. And he sees phenomenal growth in the area as it becomes interconnected with other areas of wellbeing. He believes that in the near future, the interconnected businesses of nutrition, exercise, and sleep management will evolve into a $1 trillion industry.

"It comes down to practicing certain habits," he says, "Not very complicated, but it can make a big impact in your life and how you live and how long you live. So that's how I got into Jenny Craig. Jenny Craig has been doing this for 37 years! We have a science advisory board focused on healthcare. One of the people in that advisory board is a Harvard Medical School professor. We focus on lifestyle, as well."

THE OBESITY EPIDEMIC

David believes that obesity is the number one underlying health problem in America. Obesity impairs immunity. And in a situation like Covid-19, it becomes even the most important thing.

And obesity starts when people are young, which is the time when a company like Jenny Craig can intervene and inculcate healthy habits and behaviors. Jenny Craig, with David's encouragement, has introduced an app that is designed to help teenagers educate themselves about healthy habits and eating.

"We're using gamification," David says, "but we also became more centered on e-commerce through Covid-19, and we implemented an omni-channel transformation."

LIFE PRIORITIES

David believes that when people look good and are fit, they feel more confident. It is an educational effort. After all, people can enjoy a healthy relationship with food. Food is not an enemy. He believes that food is wonderful.

Part of the Jenny Craig philosophy is centered on monitoring one's intake of both salt and sugar. Another factor is portion control, which David believes is an emotional/socialized factor. In America, he notes that many children are brought up to overeat because they are told that it is "bad" to leave uneaten portions of food on their plates. We are actually conditioned to eat everything that is put in front of us. And what are we eating? We know that the North American diet is not balanced.

"The American comfort diet is very intense on carbohydrates," David notes. "About 70 percent of it is going to be carbohydrates and the remaining 30 percent is going to be between proteins, vegetables, and certain other things. That's just an average. We learn to eat that way over time, and when we are 30, it is difficult to change those behaviors that we learned when we were kids."

Changing that requires education and assistance. So instead of just giving clients a list of foods to eat, Jenny Craig has dieticians who sit down with clients, set targets, and work with them flexibly to find what will work for them.

"I did it myself," David says. "For some people, coffee is not a problem. I have espresso but when I have the long American coffees a few times a day, basically I lose a lot of nutrients that I need to keep in my body. So having a nutritionist or having a coach that works with you can actually help you build that relationship in a healthy way."

JENNY CRAIG'S GROWING
COOPERATION WITH WALGREENS

As this book nears publication, Jenny Craig has already placed about 400 offices—each staffed by Jenny Craig counselors—in Walgreens stores.

When Walgreens customers find out that those counselors are on site, they often inquire about Jenny Craig services and counseling. After all, those customers happened to be in those Walgreens facilities anyway, so they are likely to want to stop in to see what Jenny Craig does. And after they have an initial consultation with a Jenny Craig nutritional counselor, many start to schedule further sessions—often once a week—to come back for more counseling.

David feels that the Jenny Craig philosophy of helping customers goes a long way toward cementing those relationships, ultimately helping clients establish long-running changes in their relationship with food.

"A counselor is important to help our clients understand where a problem with food is coming from," he explains. "Maybe it's coming because a client has an unhealthy relationship with his or her partner. Maybe it's rooted in the fact that a client has lost a loved one, or because it's Thanksgiving and socially, everyone is conditioned to believe they have to eat everything and more. A Jenny Craig counselor helps us understand that. What are the social pressures? What are the fears that people have? How can they develop the conviction to do certain things, to change things? So we work through the coaching. We work out a lot into how people think and on building the conviction to go after goals."

"Walgreens is really well positioned in the industry," David adds, "as your neighborhood local relationship healthcare provider, where you can find just about anything healthcare related that you need. We help you with weight loss through obesity challenges and diabetes challenges. It's a great relationship. Symbiosis between the two!"

And now Walgreens and Jenny Craig are aligned with Kroger food stores too. "The opportunity there is just incredible," David says. "And so that's really the focus at the moment. And we don't think that the goal is to have as many cooperations and opportunities as we possibly can. It's a matter of having a few very meaningful ones. And Walgreens right now is the right one. We are focused on that success. We have a symbiosis between what they do and what we do. We have millions of customers, and we work with plans to lose millions of pounds, and Walgreens also has millions of customers. I think those are great opportunities."

David is saying, and I agree, that we are driving change and convincing a growing number of people that there is an intimate, and strong, relationship between nutrition, exercise, and good health.

MEET GOMO HEALTH

Specialty meal delivery programs are emerging that provide clinically proven, evidenced-based meal plans along with digital health engagement tools to help improve risk factors for type 2 diabetes and heart disease.

Imagine—new Jenny Craig members receive prepared meals directly at their door and along with their first order a welcome kit of devices and a data hub you plug into any socket. Their biometrics are remotely tracked on blood pressure cuffs, glucometers and smart scales and the hub sends the information to an analytics platform that detects emerging problems. Negative trends are detected early so corrective measures can be taken. Upon delivery of your welcome kit, Jenny Craig's GoMo Health Concierge checks in with a text to make sure everything is all set up and offers to answer any questions. From time to time,

GoMo Concierge nudges you to make sure you are stepping on your scales and taking your other vitals. It is a data driven world and having a longitudinal view helps everyone understand how to deliver a more personalized experience.

Connecting to on-demand coaches and your care team is never more than a click away. Not everyone likes "heat and eat" meals so GoMo nudges you toward Kroger so you can also cook healthy meals at home. Virtual cooking classes come with your meal subscription.

Soon, Jenny Craig will be helping you create grocery lists, highlighting the best menu options at popular restaurants, and continuing to send tips, tricks, and educational videos to keep you motivated. GoMo will be the nudge that keeps you engaged.

The goal is to help drive and sustain behavior change so you can enjoy the results achieved. You can continue to order your prepared meals or contact your coach or clinical staff if you need a little extra support.

GOMO RESULTS FOR PEOPLE WITH CARDIOMETABOLIC DISEASE AND DIABETES

GoMo's meal programs have been shown to work, as documented by several randomized clinical trials. With 66 percent of diabetics having hypertension and 94 percent of individuals with pre-diabetes suffering from cholesterol and/or triglyceride problems, the boundaries of chronic disease are quickly blurring. EatFitGo, Mom's Meals, GA Foods and others are offering meal programs that promise to be effective in simultaneously improving multiple cardiometabolic risk factors in people suffering from multiple chronic diseases, including metabolic syndrome.

People with hypertension who take part in these programs will reduce their total cholesterol and their LDL cholesterol. They can also expect lowered systolic blood pressure by an average of 10.00 mm.

Results for people with diabetes can be just as dramatic. They have reduced fasting blood sugar, reduced HbA1c levels, and cut their triglyceride levels too.

Along the way, GoMo nudges members to lose weight and track their biometrics meticulously throughout the year. Members with diabetes are expected to lose an average of about seven pounds in the first year and members with cardiovascular disease should do even better, with an average weight loss of about 14 pounds. And people like their meals —71 percent of people stick with the program for a year and report high levels of satisfaction with their life changes.

MEET NUTRITION VISIONARY TOM RIFAI, MD

We weren't surprised that when we video chatted with Dr. Tom Rifai, he was taking a power walk through his neighborhood. Talking into his phone he stayed completely focused and on-topic every step of the way. As he walked, we got a visual tour of his neighborhood.

Tom is the primary author and online course director of Harvard's "Nutrition and the Metabolic Syndrome" program which integrates his 5 Keys to Optimal Wellness that he developed. It is one of Harvard's most popular online Lifestyle Medicine courses, attended by more than 4,000 doctors and other healthcare providers worldwide. Tom has written extensively about those 5 keys and is currently writing a book on what he calls a Flexitarian lifestyle that is based on them.

Tom, like many of the other leaders we speak with in this book, followed his own personal path to health. In his younger years, he was overweight. He didn't exercise or follow a healthy diet. Yet you would never know that now. Tom is a fit ball of high energy, and he explains the process in terms that apply both to himself and to others.

"People think once they understand nutrition and the pay-off, they will be motivated to change habits, lose weight, become healthier and enjoy other benefits," Tom says, "I prefer to see the process not as depriving ourselves of anything, but as *providing* us the opportunity to achieve our life goals. Part of it centers on budgeting foods that we eat, not depriving ourselves. I avoid the terms good and bad regarding food because they don't really mean anything.

"There's nothing technically that I would consider off the menu. It's all a matter of how often and how much you are eating, and what you are getting for the price. I would say that bargain you strike with what you eat will pay you back in the way you feel, the way you look, whether you can keep up with your grand-children, whether you can travel the Galapagos, or whether you can maintain your sexual health until you're 90. Things like that are real, not made-up. Those are real motivators that can drive someone to understand that in food choices, it is a question of providing, not depriving.

"We can't really compare a jelly bean to a navy bean," Tom adds with a laugh." I mean, they are completely different meta-bolic animals. It's not smart to consider something as just carbs and not differentiate its calorie density, its fiber, its rate of glucose release based on its molecular structure, and just say they are the same thing. Nutrition has to be filtered in a way that is sensitive to the individual. Their historical likes, dislikes, their ethnic back-ground, their family. But ultimately, it is huge. Food is huge.

"My mindset is that I am not committed to changing my diet. But I am committed to maintaining my intellectual curiosity about how people think about nutrition."

ON TREATING TYPE 2 DIABETES

Rather than focusing on diet and nutrition alone, the best approach is to address a number of issues that include not just diet but also hypertension, weight management, lipid dyslipidemia and the prevention of it. Tom believes that sleep disruption is an invitation to poor health. And exercise is another key component of good health.

"Physical movement throughout the day is a key to better health for people who have diabetes," Tom explains, "Breaking up movement throughout the day is critical, number one, in addition to exercise too. All of these are part of the cardio metabolic spectrum," Tom says.

ON TOOLS TO MEASURE HEALTH

"I would say that your smart-scale has a role to play. It's definitely convenient, but it's hardly a body composition analysis. Nevertheless, if we're looking at blood pressure, triglycerides, blood sugar, weight, that will typically tell us better than trying to give one a calorie target because it's just an impossible target to actually get right."

That statement that Tom just made seems so simple, but it is also very wise. For most of us, there are so many factors to monitor, so many dietary and other changes to make that it makes little sense to try to achieve health by fixating on only one or two of them.

The key, if you will, is making it easy and understandable to achieve.

As Tom was ending both his walk and our chat, he summed it all up in the following way.

The 5 key areas to track are:

- Psychology – "The way we think about who we are and what we eat."

- Nutrition – "We are what we eat."

- Physical activity – "I like to keep it simple but be consistent."

- Environments – "Your home, your work, your social determinants."

- Accountability—"It's your health."

Tom explains, "Those five things—psychology, nutrition, activity, environments and accountability—make up the core aspects that almost anyone who wants to go through a transformation lifestyle change process needs to understand. And those are the areas where they generally need to build their skills."

Now, let's explore another business that has a dramatically different approach to thinking about nutrition—different, but equally effective.

DISRUPTING THE DISRUPTORS: ELO HEALTH

Ari Tulla is the co-founder and CEO of Elo Health, a startup that uses AI, blood test results, and expert guidance to provide nutrition recommendations precisely calibrated to your unique needs. What is Elo Health? The company mission both teases and explains the company vision:

"Our vision is to transform food from the cause of disease to medicine."

Elo has built a ground-breaking platform that analyzes over 3,000 peer-reviewed studies, personal biomarker results, questionnaire information, and data from wearables, to take the guesswork out of food and supplement decisions.

Their first product is a supplement offering; however, they plan to expand to food in the near future. The team at Elo knows that supplements are complementary to food, rather than a standalone strategy for optimizing nutrition and, ultimately, health.

HOW ELO WORKS

Members start with a quick, at-home blood test they perform on themselves. Elo AI ingests these results, as well as questionnaire and wearable data, to build a precise micronutrient plan for each individual's needs and goals.

After this, members meet with an Elo Health Coach to review their recommendations and tweak their plan, as needed. This session gives Elo members the opportunity to ask questions and make sense of their plan.

Then, Elo sends a monthly supply of personalized supplements, separated into daily packets, straight to their door. Blood work is repeated periodically to ensure continued optimization.

"Health is dynamic, and your supplement regime should be too," according to Elo. "*We call this nutrition with precision.*"

And your Elo Health Coach doesn't just disappear after the first session. They're with you every step of the way, relentlessly optimizing your plan and supporting your health journey.

ABOUT ARI TULLA

Elo isn't Ari's first rodeo. Before Elo, Ari was the CEO of Quest Analytics. And before that, Ari was co-founder and CEO of BetterDoctor, a company dedicated to providing people with accurate data about their healthcare providers. Ari left his role at

Quest Analytics in 2019 and formed Elo in 2020 with two other seasoned entrepreneurs, Tapio Tolvanen, and Miklu Silvanto.

If you think those names sound Scandinavian, you're right. Ari, Tapio and Miklu are Finnish. Ari and Tapio met at Nokia, the Finnish mobile phone giant, founded BetterDoctor, and have been working together for over a decade. Miklu spent nearly a decade at Apple's legendary industrial design team led by Jony Ive.

Not surprisingly, the Finnish connection flows into Elo. Everything seems modern, streamlined, simplified, and somehow beautiful.

Today, Ari lives in northern California with his family. Like a true Scandinavian, he is an avid outdoorsman.

LET'S TALK WITH ARI

Are we at a point where we should think of food as simply fuel, or is it really medicine for the mind and body? Ari brings it all into focus and provides a historical perspective.

"Over the last 50 years," he observes, "we have seen obesity go from nonexistent to prevalent. About 40 percent of adults in the U.S. today are obese and it's costing trillions of dollars every year. But it's not just about the money—obesity is reducing our health span, life expectancy, and potential. We can't do great things when we're sick.

"Over the years, we've fallen in and out of love with so many food fads, which have contributed to our weight problem. In the early days, Hungry Man—a TV dinner with 5,000 calories— became big, along with Coke and other sugar bombs. Then in the 1970s and 80s, we condemned fat and removed it from everything. In parallel, we started adding sugar and high fructose corn syrup to food. Then by the late 2000s, we had this coffee movement where coffee changed from a healthy black liquid into the equivalent of a sugary soda. That added yet another layer."

THE OBESITY TREND

Ari points out that those trends, along with a reliance on ultra-processed foods, are still exacerbating the obesity epidemic today. Seventy-five percent of adults are overweight. Both Ari and I honestly believe that the food industry is poised to become the next tobacco industry in terms of how much harm their products are doing to people.

Governments worldwide are going to set their sights on the ultra-processed food manufacturers and say to them, "You knew that the product was addictive and bad for us. You knew that adding sugar to absolutely everything would lead to obesity and chronic, diet-related illnesses like type 2 diabetes."

This political dialogue will force the food industry to clean up their act, reduce sugar and think harder about their influence on population health. The cherry on top of all of this is that people are wildly confused about what's good for them, and what's bad.

"Nutrition misinformation is rife," Ari says, "and the food industry is doing its best to muddy the waters with pseudoscience. It's difficult for consumers to differentiate between snake oil and science. People are trying to get healthier and testing out new (old) eating approaches like paleo and intermittent fasting—so the interest is there—but few people know where to turn for the right advice.

"We founded Elo to provide consumers with honest, science-based answers to their nutrition questions and make nutrition science easier to understand and implement. We fundamentally believe that food can be turned from the cause of disease to medicine."

WHERE ELO FITS

Elo and its care team have been narrowing down and focusing on men age 40+, who are most likely to develop conditions like type 2 diabetes, elevated cholesterol, and high blood pressure. Interestingly, that group was the first generation to dive head-first into processed foods. Both Ari and I are part of this cohort. As kids, we ate hot dogs, hamburgers, and pizza, and later, many foods laced with sugar and high fructose corn syrup.

Ari and his team have concluded that the goal is not to build a food product or supplement. It's about building a platform that provides the right nutrition recommendations for consumers' unique needs, underpinned by science.

And then there is the longer view.

"When we think about this," Ari says, "what we are really selling is confidence about the next 30 years. I want to build a system that can help Elo members age with confidence and achieve their goals.

"Thirty years from now, I'm going to be 72. I plan to be able to do many of the things I love doing today: hiking, skiing, and taking long bike rides. I might not be as fast in 30 years' time, but if I can do those things with my kids and expand my life span and health span which is defined as years without disease, I will be happy. And that's what Elo is all about—helping you perform at your best at every age.

"One of the trickiest parts of the problem we're solving, is that there's no 'one size fits all approach' to nutrition. We know that eating a lot of plants is good for us but beyond that, what works for you and what works for me can be very different. Food is personal. It's influenced by our cultural heritage, genetic make-up, taste preferences, activity levels, biochemistry, and many other factors.

"At Elo, we start by understanding you and your body. We spend most of our time analyzing your longitudinal health record, biomarker information, activity, sleep data, and weight history. From there, we translate that data into actionable nutrition recommendations, precisely tailored to your unique needs."

Elo has a unique way of doing things. Part of the mission and philosophy is to recognize that the "human touch" is important and that there are some things that cannot be replicated by an algorithm. As Ali puts it, "We all need support to develop new habits."

A PERSONAL STORY

Ari says, "Everyone has their own time clock and their own sense of priorities. Everyone also has what I call memento mori. Memento mori is basically that moment your internal clock reminds you that 'You are mortal, you are mortal, you are mortal! Don't forget it!' Maybe this moment happens when you go to a friend's funeral for the first time, or a family member gets sick. Or perhaps you have your own health scare. Memento mori is the moment when you realize that life is finite and want to take action to preserve it. For many men, it happens in their 40s and 50s and that's exactly who we're helping at Elo.

"My memento mori moment took place in the summer of 2000. I was in London with my wife, Anu. We were having a great holiday and exploring the British Museum exhibit about ancient Egyptian art.

"Anu pressed a button on the neck of the sarcophagus and listened to a story about the common causes of death 2,000 years ago. At that time, people only lived to 39 years old and often died of thyroid tumors. As Anu listened to the story she felt her neck. Suddenly she turned at me and said, "Could you listen to this and touch my neck?" I touched her neck and felt a bump similar to that described in the audio. We got back home, and a couple of weeks later, Anu was in the operating room having a large tumor removed from her neck. At the time, Anu was 22 years old, a healthy, athletic, young woman and we had no idea that this incident would lead to tremendous changes for us both.

"Luckily, the tumor ended up being benign, however, Anu's surgery removed part of her thyroid, which led to autoimmune diseases and hormonal imbalances. Little by little we got Anu's health in check by optimizing diet, sleep, mindfulness, and exercise. We both adopted a no-wheat, no-sugar, little-meat diet that we still follow today.

"These lifestyle interventions, together with modern reproductive science, helped us get pregnant, and our two wonderful kids are proof that food is medicine."

BUILDING ACCEPTANCE
FOR THE IDEA THAT FOOD IS MEDICINE

You could argue that much of what we do in healthcare, especially from the health plan perspective, is on a conveyer belt. There is a lot of repeatable processing that just comes with the territory. We frequently cheer on the innovators because without them, health plans would largely be about processing claims.

It is when you stray outside of those core competencies that you realize a different perspective is needed for creating anything new and exciting. Sailors would say, this is when you need a seasoned skipper at the helm to navigate the nuances and complexities of the looming potential storm. Where consumerism and the regulatory process collide, you need the right blend of forward thinking and the ability to execute in the here and now. To excel and deliver real measurable value, you need to know how to pivot and learn from your mistakes.

Darrik Erikstrup is product manager at BrightHealthCare. com but he is the skipper at the helm when it comes to defining meal delivery benefits for Bright Healthcare's Medicare Advantage members. Bright Healthcare is easily one of the more innovative new plan providers, dedicated to offering customers a variety of healthcare coverage plans that are robust and reasonably priced.

Bright is not afraid of taking innovative steps to improve the health of consumers and their families too.

For example, Darrik is a big believer that food and nutrition can be a major factor in a wide variety of care-related issues. When people arrive home from the hospital, for example, the kind of food they eat plays a major role in how they recover and subsequently maintain their health. Food is, in fact, a form of medicine.

Plus, Darrik believes in assuring that a patient's entire family has access to good nutritional choices. "When someone comes home from the hospital and can't shop for healthy foods for the family," he says, "they can end up going to fast food stores and bringing home foods that are unhealthy, but pre-prepared and convenient to serve."

That's another way of saying that nutrition can play a holistic role in improving health and quality of life for a large part of the population.

You have got to admire the fact that Bright HealthCare is trying to get ahead of health-related issues and proactively taking steps to make things better by focusing on nutrition, in a larger way.

"I think from a healthcare perspective, what we are doing is not new," Darrik says. "But what is new is the receptiveness of our audience.

"Healthy food has always been available, but how do we get folks to get excited about nutrition, about eating healthily? How do we encourage people to better understand that what they eat will have a major impact on their overall well-being?

"A lot of issues of acceptance have to do with where we are as a country and even globally, about how we're thinking about food. Suddenly, food and diet are getting a lot of attention. You frequently see celebrities that are endorsing some type of raw food diet or the paleo diet, or some type of supplement that they think is changing their life.

"So, nutrition, in a way, is getting attention in the communities that folks are in and that's creating greater reception to the idea of food as medicine. People are discovering that eating right can often lead to feeling better. You're hearing a lot of stories about people with diabetes who are reporting that a healthier diet replaced the need for gastric bypass surgery and their need for costly ongoing meds. Social media and streaming platforms are helping 'Food as Medicine' get the credibility that it deserves. We seem to have developed an appetite, if you will, for information in this area."

HOW IS FOOD AS MEDICINE (FAM) EVOLVING?

Bright HealthCare has already been offering home-delivered meals to customers. But company leadership is recognizing that delivering meals isn't only about assuring that customers can keep eating to avoid hunger. Nutrition, in fact, is a vital part of recovery and maintaining good health.

"We've traditionally had a post-discharge home-delivered meals solution," Darrik says, "which is fantastic and has supported members at their most vulnerable time; when they're being discharged from the hospital and ensuring that they have nutritious meals to support recovery. Now, we are striving to expand the program by improving engagement and education. We believe our efforts will help take the awareness that food is medicine to the next level."

THE PANDEMIC'S EFFECT
ON MEAL AND FOOD DELIVERY

During the pandemic, we have seen the meal delivery market just explode. With consumers hesitant to be in contact with other people, it only made sense.

Yet Darrik points out that the safety inherent in food and meal delivery became even more important, during the pandemic, to people with health issues that place them in high-risk categories. Suddenly, having meals delivered safely home was more important than the simple convenience of fast food.

"Supporting high-risk individuals in their own homes with healthy food is a great way to exemplify being there for our members," Darrik explains. "Being able to do it while helping them minimize the risks of being out in the public is also a huge positive.

"Think about somebody who's diabetic, low income, who is getting toward the end of the month and running out of food stamps or some other type of supplemental program that's providing them access to healthy foods. Or maybe they are running low on funds and only have access to unhealthy fast foods. Having a supplement from your insurance company allows you to stay on track. That goes above and beyond and demonstrates the value that we see in maintaining a healthy diet and healthy lifestyle."

HOW WILL PROGRAMS LIKE THESE SUCCEED?

"I think that success comes down to understanding who your members are and tailoring a program based on those needs," Darrik says. "I think any time you can give members options they can relate to, you're setting up your opportunity for success.

"Look at the general Medicare population. What is their need for meal supplements? How does that differ from the needs of someone in that population who is type 2 diabetic or in a pre-diabetic stage? Because all of those require a different level of care and different nutrition and exercise plans. That is where we need to be strategic in how we are approaching food as medicine with members."

What is the best way to start delivering this extra level of care?

"I think that success depends on how you launch the program. What type of information are you trying to gain access to on the front end? Are you asking probing questions? Are you asking the right questions that are going to allow members to be successful?

"If you're telling somebody who primarily eats meat that they need to switch to a vegetarian diet, you're likely not going to see success. So, how do you set up that individual for reducing red meat intake and increasing leafy greens? You've got to approach it in a way that is going to be attractive to them.

"And I think the same is true if you are trying to help somebody manage their diabetes if they love to eat Pop-Tarts and donuts for breakfast, lunch and dinner, then you can't just say, 'From now on, it's salads with kale and carrots and that's it.' You have to offer choices that appeal while educating on cause and effect with food choices.

"It is helping people develop a long term strategy for success so they can see that the relationship they have with food can profoundly affect their overall health. And that goes back to understanding your members and helping them discover options to be successful."

Darrik is motivated by helping people be healthier. For him, this is the holy grail. You can't boldly proclaim your meal program is a success simply because people are ordering the meals— outcomes matter. Everyone benefits from thinking like this. It is when you look at this through the prism of connected health that you see the full potential of food as medicine (FAM). Imagine schools applying FAM concepts to their cafeteria menu and vending machine offerings, curriculum reinforcing the importance of nutrition as a fundamental pillar of good health and social services sending needy latch-key kids home with nutritious meals. If good nutrition becomes the new normal, we are on our way to making a difference already.

SOME FINAL THOUGHTS FROM KEVIN

We're just at the precipice of the digital health revolution and yet to unlock the true capabilities of health tools like Apple HealthKit, Oura Ring, and the Apple Watch. At Elo, we want to be part of that conversation and trailblaze a new category of health offerings that integrate data from many channels. I believe that ten years from now we will look back and think that healthcare isn't anything like it was a decade ago.

Staying healthy is complicated. It's never just one thing that you can fix. Many people are looking for a magic bullet, but it doesn't work like that. Adequate sleep, stress management, regular exercise, and wholesome nutrition work in concert, and sometimes they get out of sync.

Nutrition is arguably the trickiest to fix—we're up against powerful marketing messages, cultural beliefs, and 50 years of ultra-processed food—but that's what makes our work at Elo exciting and meaningful.

CHAPTER FIVE:

HOW SCHOOLS CONNECT TO HEALTHCARE

"Healthy children make for healthier adults."
—Andy Slavitt, Acting Administrator
of the Centers for Medicare and Medicaid Services

Let me share a few memories about what it was like to go to school when I was a kid - back in the 1960s and 70s.

Bear with me because my recollections are probably going to seem a little stereotyped. But all my rather homespun memories represent events that are actually true for me, for the very simple reason that I grew up in a rural area of Vermont.

OK, here comes the nostalgia. Did I really walk to school every day, no matter the snow or the rain or the cold? Yes, I pretty much did. Were the schools I attended at least bigger than the one-room schoolhouses that once functioned as educational buildings back in the even older days? Yes, but not by much.

Was it muddy in Vermont? Yes, and it still is today, during New England's famous "mud season." When team practice began for spring sports and it was time to do sit-ups, we actually looked for patches of snow and lay down there, because it was nicer than lying down in the mud. And did some of our teachers look like the ones that Norman Rockwell envisioned and painted—the dowager elder ladies in pale, pastel blue dresses with hair that probably resulted from using Toni home permanent wave kits that were bought at the general store? Yes, some of them did.

The reason I am writing about those olden days is not to make you pity me, but to make a point, which is that things have changed monumentally in education, and in schools, since the days when I was growing up. I am also striving to make the point that the changes that have occurred go way, way beyond changes in the optics I mention just above. One thing is that most of the people in rural areas of our country are now going to big, modern regional high schools, not the high school on the hill, and that is certainly different. I am talking about profound functional and operational philosophical changes in what we now expect from our schools, and in what they deliver.

SCHOOLS AREN'T WHAT THEY USED TO BE

Here is a top-of-mind list of ways that our schools have changed, with an emphasis not only on the educational product they produce but on social and societal changes as well.

Hours have been extended – When I was growing up, the school day ended at about 3:00 PM, with the exception of the days when I had athletic practices to attend, or the occasional club meeting. Back in the days before in-classroom STEM studies, there used to be chemistry clubs, physics clubs, and even math clubs that met after school. There were French clubs and Latin clubs too. Today, school days are longer. Schools keep kids in study halls, in tutoring, and in all kinds of extra-hours activities that last until dinner time. In some cases, I suspect, this change has occurred because there are far more households in which both parents are working, and they need schools to care for kids for more hours every day. Another reason is the growth in the number of single-parent households in America. Schools have taken on an increased role that might be loosely called childcare. One result is that schools play a greater role in the socialization of children than ever before.

Schools provide meals for more and more students – OK, here is a big change. We have arrived at a point in history when many families rely on schools to feed their children. Who could have seen that one coming? In many school systems, school-provided breakfasts are the first source of nutrition that students have at the start of the day. Some schools not only go on to provide lunch, but dinner as well. This is a major factor not only in how well-fed our nation's children are, but in how well educated they are too. Kids who are hungry, or who are malnourished, simply do not learn well. In a very real sense, our schools' ability to provide nutrition determines our future as a nation. A better-educated country, we know, is better equipped to succeed, and compete in international trade.

Schools are now remote educators – Thanks to the Covid-19 pandemic, our schools have become quite adept at offering education remotely to their students. They are offering virtual courses that could compete in scope and content to those that were being used at colleges and universities only a few years ago. And now that schools have learned to teach in this way – and now that students and their families have started to accept a newly hybridized learning model that combines classroom and remote learning – it seems likely that this new way of learning will come to be permanently used in our schools. It works, we are learning how to do it, it can be economically delivered, and it promises still more benefits. Why wouldn't our schools continue to use it?

Schools are playing a bigger role in social and healthcare outreach – In poorer metro areas, school officials are often the front line that knows when kids are experiencing a number of problems, from chronic diseases or a lack of cleanliness, to not getting required vaccinations, to psychological problems, and even to domestic disruption and violence. Of course, schools played some of this role when I was a kid growing up. If one of my classmates showed up with a black eye or was hungry or seemed to have not slept for a few days, someone in the school administration would step in and ask why. But the primary role of our schools was to educate kids. I would mention reading, writing and 'rithmetic, but perhaps that is taking my nostalgia too far.

TALKING WITH AUSTIN BEUTNER ABOUT ONE OF THE MOST MODERN SCHOOL SYSTEMS IN AMERICA

Austin Beutner is superintendent of the Los Angeles Unified School District, a position he has held since 2018.

The moment you begin to talk with Austin about education, you sense immediately that he is a man who has a deep and genuine commitment to both education and children's wellbeing. You also learn that he pursued a unique path as he matured into those core beliefs. Austin, who grew up in Michigan, attended Dartmouth College in New Hampshire. His mother was a schoolteacher, and his father was an engineer—a duality that could account for both his interest in children and in creating well-run structures that support them. His success in a number of different fields also led him to where he is now. He previously was the publisher and CEO of the *Los Angeles Times* and the *San Diego Union-Tribune*, which helps explain how he developed a keen insider's knowledge of education in California and Los Angeles. He also served as deputy mayor of Los Angeles in 2011 and 2012, and actually entered the race to become mayor of Los Angeles before other priorities led him to set aside that plan.

"When we look at all the intersect points with healthcare," Austin says, "we see that we have largely ignored how influential our schools can be in healthcare. With that as the backdrop, let's start the conversation around the value of nutrition and explore how schools can better teach kids the importance of eating and eating properly. That's an area where schools could do better. Let me reframe Andy Slavitt's statement about how healthy children make healthier adults and tell you that from my perspective, healthier children make better learners. The intersection of health and school-based health has been one of the missing pieces in our society.

"I want to just share a life example from something I've been working on for many years, which I think illustrates something different about our vision for our children. But before we get to the hierarchy of needs, before we get to informing about nutrition, we have to make sure nutrition is available. If you look at what we're doing in this pandemic, we have now provided more than 85 million meals to students and families throughout the Los Angeles area. But 80 percent of the families we serve were living in poverty before the pandemic.

"And to give you some perspective, we serve a population with a median household income of $22,000 in Los Angeles. That's household income, not individual. And now, we estimate that as many as three-quarters of the families we serve have lost work through the pandemic. And we're not serving meals at every school, even though we are serving into each region. During the pandemic, we have started food relief efforts at 63 additional schools. We've also provided diapers and other needed supplies.

"Before we start talking about the value of nutrition, we need to address food insecurity and the fact that very basic needs are not being met. I could take you into one of our schools, so you can see how we provide breakfast in classrooms. And you will see that a meaningful number of our students are clearly hungry. It's clear they haven't had nutrition since they were last in school. And you can see it in their response because you can tell if a child is hungry. So, before we get to educating children on the value of nutrition, we have to be making sure food is available at all. That is our greater challenge at the moment, although we can talk about upgrading from a muffin to carrots or whatever, about the hierarchy of better food. And by the way, we do a lot of work in schools to make sure we are providing the healthiest possible set of meals.

"We do all kinds of focus groups. That just means our folks who manage our school lunch program go to schools and listen to kids. Students will tell you what they'll eat. Now, the question is, you have to find an intersection between what's healthy and what they'll eat, and then build the value of nutrition."

SCHOOL-BASED HEALTHCARE

In addition to shouldering responsibility for making school-delivered meals both more appealing and more nutritious, Austin and his team at the board of education are undertaking a number of programs to support school children and their families. For eight years now, they have been involved with Vision to Learn, an organization that provides free school-distributed eyeglasses to kids in low-income communities. "If a student cannot see the board, that student is just not going to be in the game," Austin observes, and notes that as many as 25 percent of school children in Los Angeles have eyesight limitations that are probably limiting their ability to learn.

Thanks to the success that Vision to Learn programs achieved in Los Angeles, they are now being used in 350 cities across the United States. Austin points to research conducted at Johns Hopkins University that shows that programs that improve students' ability to see represent the most powerful and effective kind of classroom interventions. Interestingly, programs that target eyesight are turning out to have an even larger effect on student learning than are programs that improve students' access to technology.

"It's intuitively obvious that students who have vision problems will be struggling," Austin says. He adds that vision problems can be a barometer that can lead to the detection of other health problems in children. "When going to a juvenile detention center, children from low-income families that are having their vision checked are often getting the first physical exam they've had in their lives," he adds, "or maybe since they left the hospital when they were born. In Texas, 70 percent of kids who enter the system have uncorrected vision issues. You can see it. Kids who get glasses do better. Kids who don't get glasses, as early as kindergarten, get misdiagnosed as having behavior problems. By fourth grade, they're mislabeled as slow learners.

By eighth grade, they drop out and not much later, they're part of the juvenile detention system."

Austin's point is incredibly powerful. Schools accurately—and often unfortunately—reflect the health and well-being of the communities they serve, whether it's in nutrition, in eye care, in access to a wider array of services. Yet schools are also uniquely positioned to help.

COVID-19 TESTING IN SCHOOLS

"We're providing free Covid-19 testing at schools," Austin states. "Think a little bit about that. And we've got this tremendous consortium of partners helping us. We've now done more of that testing, I think, than any other school system in the world does. We are talking about a few hundred thousand students and staff, and we see huge disparities in the willingness of families to take part, to have their child come get a free test. In more affluent communities, we've now got 25 percent participation in similar Covid-19 testing programs. But in low-income communities, only five to six percent participate."

Austin and his team have undertaken studies, and conducted focus groups, to try to understand why lower-income families are more reluctant to have their children tested for Covid-19. "Pretty quickly," Austin states, "we can see a group of six or seven people in a small testing room, maybe an unheated room where the people who have come to be tested are from multiple generations.

"They are concerned that that their 10-year-old child will bring the virus home to grandma—a grandma who gets sick and frequently without access to adequate healthcare. They don't want to know if they're asymptomatic because they feel OK, and they need to go to work because work is essential to put a roof over their heads, and food on the table. And they don't trust government.

"So that's the long-winded answer. But in many, many communities, adequacy is the first issue before you can get to the message about better nutrition."

STRUCTURAL CONSIDERATIONS IN BETTER MEAL DISTRIBUTION IN SCHOOLS

The issues that Austin is telling us about are sobering problems. Finding solutions to them is hindered by what I would call the "siloed" nature of healthcare. If you look at Los Angeles, you see that there's a city, a county, a school district, and they all operate separately from a governance structure. They each have separately elected officials, separate administrative teams.

Austin explains, "So of the meals we've provided—85 million meals—about 30 million have gone to adults. The other 55 to children. Those children may or may not be in our schools; we ask no questions. You could be documented or undocumented. You could be in our schools, or not in our schools. We feed you. We provide 85 million meals.

"We're doing it because we saw an unmet need. We saw the hungry families. We said, OK, we're going to try to address that. You look in terms of connecting—the computers and the internet access that needs to go with that. About a quarter of the families we serve have no computers or internet access, because the inadequacy of funding for education. And we have large class sizes, school libraries without librarians. One of the other symptoms of inadequacy would be the lack of computer devices for every child. We had to invest in those, and we had to actually secure the broadband so that we could provide it to the child in their family for free. We pay something for it. Again, that's a systemic problem that as school districts we've had to solve that wasn't solved by the city.

"You might be old enough to remember when everyone had a rotary phone. There were no haves and have nots. Everyone had one. And the system was set up to make sure that those who couldn't afford it still had it. They were connected. Somehow, we went to wireless and broadband, at least in Los Angeles. A quarter of families that we serve aren't connected. We simply had to make sure they got connected in a hurry."

WHAT WILL BREAK DOWN THE WALLS AND GET PEOPLE TO PARTICIPATE IN HEALTH-RELATED PROGRAMS?

From his reality-based, on-site perspective, Austin sees a practical solution, which is to more fully utilize schools themselves as communications hubs within their communities. He points out that in Los Angeles, public education is already the foundation of the community. Most people live within just a few blocks of public schools. .

"What better way to deliver services to the community than the place their children are at almost every day?" Austin asks. "People trust schools to deliver nutrition, eyeglasses, Covid-19 tests, access to internet."

Yet, Austin points out, the pandemic has made some problems more visible, and therefore perhaps more likely to be addressed. Austin summarizes these issues as a "lack of connectedness in the system." But perhaps as the pandemic has upped the stakes for failure, things could soon improve.

Austin summarizes, "I'm an accidental superintendent. Ten years ago, I was deputy mayor of Los Angeles. I guess 12 years ago I was CEO of a public company. And five years ago, I was publisher of the *L.A. Times*. But when the pandemic came, it accelerated some of our strategies and the fact that we needed to support the students and families and take the lead. If others weren't going to get there with us, we were not going to wait for the cavalry or someone else to present us with the solution. We in education had to do it.

"In the state of California, there are 1,037 school districts. Covid and the health risk it represents is essentially the same in all of them. Yet there are 1,037 different approaches to the health and well-being of a school community. We don't do that for tuberculosis. Every adult gets tested before they can come on campus. Measles, mumps vaccinations are required for children. Now, somehow, we've entered this crisis with 1,037 different standards. How far apart are the desks? You wear a mask, you don't wear a mask, should you be tested? Again, we believe testing is vital. The head of the World Health Organization told us back in March the way to get control of the virus was to test, test, test so you can identify and isolate quickly. For some reason, that prescription hasn't reached our country or our state at the level it needs to. We're the only school district in the state doing it and we believe it's appropriate. And we now see from our data, children and adults can get the virus. Some of the mythology about, well, kids don't get it simply isn't true. And so even some of the narrative about, well, who do you test? Do you need to just test the staff?"

SCHOOLS AS FITNESS HUBS

Students in the Los Angeles schools have gym classes. In fact, Austin points out that often, schools are about the only reliable supporters of exercise that are available to kids. And of course, physical fitness is critical to achieving good health. Just eating well will not get the job done.

But there is a problem. During school days, outdoor playing fields and open areas around schools are accessible to students, even during after school hours when they are not in class. The problem? Those same outdoor areas are generally closed off and locked on days when schools are closed.

That does not make much sense. If schools are to do a better job of supporting fitness initiatives, they need to make their grounds open. But Austin and his team are aware of this problem, and they are working to solve it.

BEST PRACTICES GET SHARED

Austin points out that his school district and New York City's—the two biggest school systems in the country—talk to each other and share best practices and solutions. For example, Los Angeles shares insights on how they have worked with Microsoft and Apple to build information systems that are used in schools. At the moment, these systems are used to track student attendance. But their architecture will allow the systems to be adapted to monitor administration of the Covid-19 vaccine among students.

So as the pandemic recedes, students will be supported to avoid infection, stay healthy, and get back to learning. As we have pointed out, "Healthy students make for healthy adults." I think we can glean from what Austin has told us, our students are now staying healthy as they grow toward adulthood and that is incredibly encouraging.

Now, let's discover what is taking place in another major California metro area—San Francisco. Student nutrition and health are top concerns there too. But because San Francisco does things differently from other cities, it's worth understanding what is happening there. Let's hear from the person who is directing initiatives—and providing leadership.

MEET STEVON COOK

Stevon Cook served as president of the San Francisco Board of Education. He was elected to the Board of Education in November 2016.

As we have just learned, Austin Beutner pursued a rather circuitous route on his way to assuming leadership of the Board of Education in Los Angeles. Stevon's route to leadership was somewhat roundabout too. He is a fourth-generation San Franciscan and graduate of the city's public schools. But he attended Williams College in Massachusetts, where he majored in American Studies and got involved in various entrepreneurial and social impact ventures. After graduating, he returned to San Francisco where he has worked in education, politics, and business.

STEVON ON THE ROLE SCHOOLS PLAY IN FOSTERING STUDENTS' HEALTH AND WELLNESS

Stevon thinks that schools are the milieu where students develop healthy life patterns. Yet he also believes that larger "circumstances" determine childhood health.

"Research highlights that circumstances can play a big role in determining how young people are becoming unhealthy," he says. "Many problems are perpetuating from home. And people are making decisions because of the unhealthy communities they come from. And that is compounded by nutritional options within the community.

"How can schools help entire communities remain healthy? They're mostly focused on nutrition because at schools, we can control the lunch. We have PE built into the calendar as a way to promote mobility. Kids need to run around. They have a lot of energy. if I were working in any administration, I would consider whether schools can be the best leverage point for the improved care for communities."

Stevon points out that the challenge is that schools need to simultaneously address a number of different health-related issues.

"Schools can start to think about all of their practices in preventative ways, especially schools where we see poor health indicators in high concentration," Stevon states. "We see them in every incoming kindergarten class which is going to face similar challenges. That is why we have an achievement gap that hasn't moved in 40 years. We know the schools where the problems are going to be most pervasive. The achievement gap hasn't changed. Those poor health outcomes aren't changing. We know the sites where those issues will likely be elevated. What we haven't done is align our staffing to address those issues at the level necessary to see some progress."

WHAT DOES PROGRESS LOOK LIKE?

How do you move the needle? San Francisco's schools have nurses and social workers because it is a city that believes in those services. The city also has wellness centers in schools that focus on both physical and mental health.

Yet nonetheless, Stevon believes that San Francisco schools are not evaluating student health in ways that are meaningful enough.

"When families come in to enroll their kids in school," Stevon states, "we need to be able to do an intake that screens for common health issues that we know are a problem in our community. You know what they are: asthma, heart disease, diabetes, obesity, they are as common as the sunrise with every new class. We know what we're going to see, but what will we do then?

"There's a way to think about healing that is proactive and engaging and loving, and it doesn't have to be about medication and surgery, it doesn't have to be like that. I am talking about positioning schools to have preventative services and to work with families in an ongoing way, and with the cultural understanding and comfort to know how to work with those families."

ON COMMUNITY RESOURCES AND HEALTH

People develop routines and live according to behavioral patterns, no matter where they live. They shop in certain stores, visit certain parks, and favor certain activities. "That's the way a community flows," Stevon says. "This is where we get our Chinese food, this is where we buy our groceries, this is where we get our sundries. There's a flow to a community and it's ingrained. We need an approach that looks like that, one that's ongoing and can be measured. And then we can understand the flow of the community and have the cultural competency to be effective as we improve community health."

CURRENT SYSTEMIC PROBLEMS

Stevon says, "In schools, we don't really test for health. We just don't have those measurements. Based on our experience working in a community, we can see health issues.

"But that's not something that we report on to the school board annually, like we report the rate of obesity. What we've done has been focused mostly on nutrition. We have our leverage point and say, OK, we're going to have nutrition guidelines, and where we serve food that has to meet certain guidelines. We know that if these guidelines are met, kids are getting healthy options. OK, that is progress. But as a city, we haven't said that we are going to report on the health of students. We just said we're going to introduce services where we can.

"In the curriculum and in our health courses, units are focused on nutrition. But we know the community doesn't live it."

ON SCHOOL MEALS

As was the case in Los Angeles, Stevon and his team stopped serving "cardboard pizza" in their cafeterias. They stopped serving chocolate milk too. But Stevon asks what is possibly a more important question . . . what can they do in the classroom, and in school culture, to bring about improvements in the way kids eat?

"One of the issues we were having was the kids didn't like the healthy options," Stevon says. "They were throwing away healthier foods. A few options were popular and the rest, they threw out or didn't touch. I've had a lot of battles with our students and our food vendors, based on those behaviors we have observed and the feedback we have been getting. What I didn't want to have happen was for students to develop an association between bad-tasting food and healthy, which we feared was happening."

DOES BETTER SCHOOL NUTRITION LEAD DIRECTLY TO BETTER HEALTH?

Most people assume that kids will track straight toward being healthier if you offer them healthier school meals. Stevon has a certain innate knack for citing past assumptions like that and insisting on understanding what is really taking place.

"Our district has all but banned sugar," he says, "but that doesn't mean that our kids are healthier, because of all the other factors that we have mentioned."

Yet progress is being made. "The situation is definitely better than it was when I was a student," Stevon observes, "better than it was 10 years ago too. We do a better job of talking about offering healthy food, introducing what it means to have more nutritious options. We have conversations with students. We have food banks that provide healthy options, which our low-income families are adopting.

"It's about the way that people develop socially, emotionally, and mentally, and how negative emotions and situations drive compulsive behavior that may be self-destructive.

"It's like, how do you prevent alcoholism? You can diagnose it, but what do you do about it? In reality, we may need to arrive at healthier outcomes by going well beyond just food and exercise.

"The model doesn't necessarily work for the context that schools operate in. But when people opt into a lifestyle, and they have a supportive community around a specific goal, you see gains, because of the way the community is set up. You can gamify it. There's an interesting book called *Stick with It* [by Sean D. Young – ed.] that talks about the habits of behavior change, which usually create success. In terms of using technology to drive results in schools, I think if there was a way to create a game around it, the kids would be interested.

"I'm big into the technology space, but I'm one of the people that think that kids have too much access to technology. I think this is developing a dependency that is unhealthy. I think a lot of adults also struggle with technology addiction. And there are some adverse effects that people are having, especially with social media. I didn't play video games like a lot of boys do. But games, I think, could be a powerful way to get people excited about doing things related to health."

STEVON ON HIS BACKGROUND

"I was born and raised in San Francisco and attended the public schools here. I was raised with my grandparents in a historically black neighborhood called Western Addition to Fillmore. And a lot of my early influences were focused on service and being engaged. In my family, we had an annual Black History Month dinner on the last Saturday every February and all the kids had to memorize speeches. It was like an oratory contest. And I would memorize Martin Luther King's speeches.

"We grew up with this focus on communicating, being involved, and improving our community. I went to a high school in Bayview-Hunters Point that was sending a lot of students of color to college, but the high school community was decimated because of Board of Education policy, and I went back to the school soon after college and got motivated by the problem. I was excited and driven to see if I could improve the city at a policy level. I have learned a lot.

"I honestly think that we have to focus on the parents and the families and do that in a way that's culturally competent. I'm not a huge fan of putting a lot of restrictions on people. But I do think that as we look at the way communities are laid out and how food options are given to people, it's pretty screwed up. We need to do something to connect to those issues."

"How do you prop the culture shift, where people feel motivated to stop doing something that is detrimental? I think the anti-smoking cigarette campaign is a good example. It is now not cool to smoke. I stopped smoking a long time ago because mostly it was society that had shifted."

DEEP COMMUNITY COMMITMENT
AND CONNECTIONS

I have been reassured by my conversations with both Austin and Stevon.

Yes, healthier kids make for healthier adults. And maybe our society still has a long way to go. But when individuals like Austin and Stevon care so deeply about children and education, that can only mean that our children, and our society as well, are on a path to greater wellness and wellbeing.

CHAPTER SIX
THE POLITICS OF HEALTHCARE

Prior to Covid-19, many of us believed that the federal government in Washington, D.C, was the branch of government that had the most control over Americans' access to treatment and care. But when it came time to turn our attention to getting tested for Covid—and even more so, when it was time to get vaccinated—a lot of us discovered that the states where we lived, and even our counties and municipalities, were the players we had been overlooking.

We learned this lesson sometimes when we were in touch with friends and relatives who lived in other parts of the country. We would ask, "Have you gotten your test or vaccination?" and the answers we heard surprised us. Some of our friends were going to hospitals for tests. To get our shots, some were going to decommissioned Sears stores, or even to Disney theme parks. Some of us were dealing with county governments, others with state governments. In a lot of cases, we didn't know where to direct our questions.

And when it came to dealing with the "front end," in the form of websites where we could book our tests and shots, we had very different experiences. A friend of mine who lives in New Jersey reports that every aspect of scheduling his vaccinations was handled "beautifully" on a website that was created by the government of the county where he lives. A friend of mine who lives in the Los Angeles area—well, not so much.

But one thing was certain – we weren't calling Washington to ask where we could get tested or vaccinated for Covid. No, the supervision over the most troubling healthcare crisis of our lifetimes was being handled almost literally in our own back yards, and that was often surprising to many of our fellow citizens.

It might interest you to know that I actually began working on this chapter, and interviewing experts on the politics of healthcare, even before the pandemic began. It might also interest you to learn that some of the insights I gained from our thought leaders even though I spoke with them before the Covid pandemic, are about the same as what they will tell you now. That is probably because they are very smart, well-informed people who already had a grasp of the big issues and the big picture even before the virus struck.

The overriding lesson is that while our president, senators and other Washington influencers seem to be in control of our healthcare, it is more often people in our states who make the decisions and who, in the end it turns out, actually care quite personally and deeply for us.

LET'S HEAR THE VIEWS OF SENATOR BILL FRIST, M.D.

Is it possible to improve access to healthcare while reducing cost and improving the quality of care – all at the same time?

I am not the first person to define these goals. In fact, they were originally identified as The Triple Aim of Healthcare by Don Berman at the Institute for Healthcare Improvement, a Boston-based nonprofit with the stated mission to assure that people everywhere have access to the best possible care. Since then, the "Triple Aim" has become the holy grail for what vibrant healthcare should look like worldwide.

According to Senator Bill Frist, M.D., the goal of achieving the Triple Aim is both desirable and attainable. Senator Frist is one of the most distinguished public servants ever to have worked in the Senate.

He began his career as a pioneering heart and lung transplant surgeon and founded the Vanderbilt Multi-Organ Transplant Center. He then entered politics, served as a U.S. Senator for two terms, and was U.S. Senate Majority Leader. Now that he has returned to private life, Senator Frist has become an active investor in healthcare companies. His activities reflect the simple principle that one way to achieve the Triple Aim is to support and cultivate the most innovative healthcare companies, with a focus on those with the greatest potential to deliver quality care to underserved populations. He is a founding partner of Frist Cressey Ventures and Chairman of the Distinguished Executives Council of Cressey & Company. We are grateful for his insights and perspective.

"I spent 20 years in medicine doing some of the most innovative procedures at that time in medicine," Senator Frist says. "They were heart transplants, lung transplants, combined heart-lung transplants, and artificial heart left ventricular assist devices. I wanted to be the very best transplant surgeon I could possibly be.

"The Vanderbilt Multi-Organ Transplant Center, which is fifteen miles from where I live, is now home to the largest heart transplant program in the world. It does today more heart transplants than any other center in the United States. I spent about 10 years first founding then building that program. The aim was to cultivate new technologies and new transplant surgical procedures that very few people had done or seen previously. In the early 1980s only a handful of centers were doing more than 10 heart transplants, and few were attempting lung or combined heart-lung transplants. Artificial hearts were in their infancy."

Senator Frist is a thoughtful man who also had specific goals he wanted to achieve in politics. Among the topics we discussed were his motivation for spending two terms in the U.S. Senate. Driving him was a desire to improve access to quality healthcare for America's underserved populations. While in the Senate, he was a force behind formulating and passage of The Medicare Prescription Drug, Improvement, and Modernization Act of 2003, which set the benchmark/framework/competitive-bidding process -- also called the +Choice plan that became Medicare

Advantage plans. Senator Frist told me that he and Senator Edward Kennedy worked together behind closed doors to write and negotiate the bill. I am not sure how widely known that is.

"I spent 12 years in the policy world where a priority was to afford access to affordable, convenient, quality care and to address health inequities," he explains. "At that time, Medicare Advantage had only enrolled about five million people."

Currently, about 28 million Americans are enrolled in Medicare Advantage.

"HIV AIDS was another important global problem at the time, hollowing out societies around the world and claiming more than three million lives annually" Senator Frist says, "As Majority Leader and the only physician in the Senate, I, working closely under President Bush's leadership, led Senate passage of this monumental legislation which ultimately changed the course of history.

"All that innovation pulled people together in ways they never had come together before, around affordable, convenient access in an equitable approach to high-quality care. We know that in general, care in any sense has a lot of inequities built into it. But at the same time, innovation and technology made it possible to move healthcare forward.

"For the last 14 years in private life, I put all that together and began to build healthcare companies, focusing on tech-enabled health services and starting in the mid-market private investment world."

Clearly, Senator Frist views investing in and starting new healthcare companies as a way to move healthcare as a whole toward that vaunted Triple Aim. In support of that goal, he co-founded Frist Cressey Ventures.

"I'm a partner and founder," he says. "On the one hand, with Cressey and Company we take ideas at the mid-market level, and build better systems, so we can take them to scale nationally. In the venture capital or start-up world, Frist Cressey Ventures focuses on IP-enabled [Internet Protocol-enabled] health services to address in a very mission-driven way the inequities, the gaps in our healthcare system, that government with its blunt hand, just cannot address."

Senator Frist is also actively engaged in humanitarian and philanthropic outreach, including board service on the Robert Wood Johnson Foundation and The Nature Conservancy, and mission trips around the world. His commitment is nothing short of inspiring. His combination of governmental, business, and humanitarian initiatives demonstrates how much difference can be made by one committed individual. He surrounds himself with like-minded individuals equally committed to making a difference.

Where does Senator Frist see his brand of committed, humanitarian healthcare going in the future?

"A lot of the innovation we did, like unraveling the genetic code as part of the Human Genome Project - came in two years ahead of schedule, and way under a budget which was $7 billion; in the end, it probably cost $4 billion. It created the platform for much of what we call the synthetic biology revolution. Almost all the companies I get involved with today depend on that sort of digital evolution, revolution, enablement, and empowerment in some way. In my investment group, we address productivity, inefficiencies, gaps in healthcare, gaps in delivery, administration, back office, productivity, reaching patients where they are."

SPEAKING WITH D.J. WILSON
FROM STATE OF REFORM

Few experts can give us a valid overall view of what has happened in the last decade than D.J. Wilson, CEO of an organization called State of Reform.

The State of Reform, which is headquartered in Washington state, is a nonprofit organization dedicated to the mission of bridging the gap between healthcare and public policy, reporting on 15 states and federal health policy. If you want to know what is taking place in healthcare just about anywhere in the U.S., these are the people to ask.

The goal of State of Reform is to create a safe space where the public and private sectors can engage and learn from one another. Much of the need for that kind of communication resulted from the Affordable Care Act, which D. J. states has defined our last decade of health policy and health politics. That bill was so vast that in many cases, people couldn't even agree on what was in it. The result was a conversation about topics like death panels (which, of course, were never part of the bill) that dominated discussion the early part of the decade.

Hospitals thought that certain issues were addressed in the bill. Pharma had a different set of assumptions. And State of Reform stepped into the breach and endeavored to start a forum where all the different concerned entities could come into the room together and communicate and try to figure things out.

When that process began, State of Reform started a website, and then a newsletter, and then launched a series of conferences and forums to facilitate the process.

D.J. uses an analogy to explain that process. "We tried to create a safe table where people could assemble. To use Wayne Gretzky's metaphor, people needed to understand where the puck was going, so all players could try to get to that place first and decide what to do about it. It's better to know that than to know where the puck is now—that's a metaphor of what we're trying to do."

THE MACRO TRENDS AS D.J. SEES THEM

"Healthcare is an industry that is the most dependent on government regulation of any sector in America, even the defense sector. Boeing can still go sell to Malaysia or Saudi Arabia, but your hospital or health plan can't leave its local market.

"Because of the money, the politics and a lot of other reasons, there is regulation and oversight. There's public information all over the place. We can track that through relationships, but also because of what we call open-source intelligence gathering; we're just reading all kinds of info and trying to make heads or tails of it."

CREATING A COMMON LANGUAGE FOR DISCOURSE

Healthcare, for better or for worse, is a field where people use different words to refer to the same thing. Medicaid is one example. If you mention Medicaid to a group of low-income patients, they might know it as the safety net that keeps them out of poverty. If you say Medicaid to specialty physicians, they might look down their noses at it, as a low-paying reimbursement. And if you mention Medicaid to an insurance company, that will mean a very different thing all together.

That confusion began early, in what turned out to be a once-in-a-generation experience in 2009 and 2010, as Congress debated what became the Affordable Care Act. There was discussion in the Senate Finance Committee in 2009 about what a universal coverage package might look like, what single payer coverage might look like.

"There was a wide range of considerations early on in the second quarter of 2009," D.J. says. "Ultimately, we saw that the public option didn't even get out of Congress. They couldn't even agree on that, much less single payer, or universal coverage. So what does all that mean? It really depends on who you ask.

"The world over, I think people can agree that access to care is important. But access to quality and affordable care is the holy grail. It really doesn't matter whether it's a public system or a private system. I don't think that people with diabetes ultimately care who's paying their bills. They want a doctor that's focused on outcomes and not necessarily just getting to see more patients so she can bill more.

"I think the biggest threats to any policy reform are how the institutional and structural incentives align with the *status quo*. If you work your entire career in healthcare and never move outside of your silo and never stick your head up and never call for significant change, you will probably be very successful anyway."

But will that kind of self-centered process result in better care for individual consumers of healthcare services? D.J. doesn't think so, and neither do I.

HOW DO TELEHEALTH AND VIRTUAL CARE CHANGE THAT DYNAMIC?

D.J. believes that telehealth offers a new way for consumers to experience care. But he adds, "I think telehealth is an interesting example of where policy and politics meet the contextual moments."

And he offers an additional opinion that I haven't heard from many others since I have been writing about digital health. He says we shouldn't be surprised if telehealth goes away, and very quickly. One reason he believes that might happen is that the current Covid-19 contextualized environment, and allied trends, are about to change. "Obviously, the context of us staying at home is the key point," he tells me. "But for instance, CMS [Centers for Medicare and Medicare Services] is allowing audio-only telehealth to be reimbursed. And that has created all kinds of issues for your patient if you are a caregiver. Now I can pick up a smartphone and talk to my doctor and my doctor can get reimbursed for it through Medicare or Medicaid, and the commercial market has followed suit. That's really meaningful and meets the moment. You're going to see whole swaths of the marketplace no longer provide telehealth and no longer seek telehealth."

Another factor that D.J. cites is that we are trending toward a time when insurance companies will offer identical, or very similar, reimbursement models, regardless of whether a member sees a caregiver face-to-face, or via a telehealth visit on a computer or a phone.

"That's often because states are requiring it," he explains. "But that's really powerful. And in a place like Texas where a Blue Cross plan there has decided to withdraw this parity and no longer pay telehealth, you're going to see a quick erosion of that service line."

In essence, D.J. is saying that telehealth is here now because of policy and financial parity in the context of care. And that situation might not continue indefinitely.

ON TELEHEALTH IN RURAL AND REMOTE MARKETS

Something really subtle is happening. For some providers, particularly rural providers, telehealth is the only care option. So far, everybody has kind of had to embrace it—there is no choice.

But here's some context. D.J. notes, "Historically, based on research we've done some time ago and which we saw confirmed by other sources, the most important decision a person makes when picking his or her physician is the proximity to his or her house.

"And then after people make that decision, they then say, 'I chose that doctor because she is really good.' There is some self-justification.

"Some clinics aren't too excited about telehealth. They know that part of their value is that they're embedded in their communities. And if you take that away, you eliminate a primary reason why people choose that clinic over others. Likewise, health plans, justifiably or maybe unjustifiably, have concerns about fraud in relation to telehealth. We've seen some physicians who are billing codes that really can't be provided in a telehealth setting."

ON END-USER'S BELIEF
IN THEIR PRIMARY CARE PROVIDERS

Watching the trends, D.J. notices that younger, more digitally fluent people don't value strong, long-lasting relationships with their providers as much as their parents did. They like telehealth in practice and might be comfortable using it more throughout their lives.

But attitudes of older consumers are somewhat different. They want the "best" care for their family members and tend to argue in favor of in-person care. In D.J.'s experience, that belief that in-person care is simply better can be observed in other contexts too.

In support of that view, he points out that older Americans rarely change their primary care providers. Usually, they only switch a few times during their lives, and usually, only when they move. And that kind of allegiance mitigates against telehealth and its underlying structure of moving quickly from one caregiver to another.

D.J. ON DISCREPANCIES OF CARE

He points out that there are aspects to the consumer-provider relationship that transcend the issues of telehealth vs. face-to-face care.

"If caregivers are dismissive of what people are telling them, that leads to poor outcomes on the provider side," he states. "Serena Williams is a perfect example. If one of the most powerful athletes, one of the richest women in the world, can almost die because her doctors were not listening to her and they were dismissing what she was saying while she was delivering her baby, it can happen to anybody, especially to people unlike Serena –who don't have means.

"Let's put this in a different perspective. If you were to send your spouse or your mom or your dad or child into the hospital, would you trust them to go there on their own? No way. You know you've got to go in there and advocate for them."

As D.J.'s words imply, we can't trust well-meaning people who are working in a bad system. We have to create a system that is operating on the highest possible level.

ON VALUE-BASED CARE

We all talk about value-based care. The question is always, to whom are those payments made and where does the value go? In California, for instance, a lot of provider groups are paid on a capitation rate, which is sort of one definition of value, where the consumer assumes all the risk. And on the opposite side, if an insurer can keep people healthy, it can make a bigger profit.

"The flipside of that is if you keep everybody out of your office and out of the hospital, you don't take care of anybody!" D.J. points out. "You can make a nice profit until the whole thing comes crashing down in a couple of years. So, the definition of value depends on what we're really paying for and who is paying. Where does it stop? Because even in that setting where you have capitation payments from the plan to the provider groups, individual doctors are still generally paid on a fee-for-service basis."

D.J. ON POLITICS AND THE BIG QUESTIONS

"In healthcare," D.J. states, 'we're generally a mile deep and an inch wide. We're compensated. We're hired. We're educated to be specialists. In politics, we're a mile wide and an inch deep. We're elected by knowing a little bit about a lot of things. In politics, the goal is to get through a 30-second soundbite in front of any audience. As a politician, it's very hard to be the expert on healthcare, even if you are an expert politically. You might have two minutes of content, or you might have five minutes of content. Either way, it has to resonate in a memorable way and that often results in a soundbite or slogan that creates an expectation it simply cannot meet.

"When you're talking about healthcare, there's not a lot of content there after five or 10 minutes. If you are a politician, there's a disincentive to engage on healthcare because you will never look like the smartest person in the room talking about it." In fact, people tune out over too much detail preferring instead to believe that pulling a single lever will cure everything. This is the magic wand approach.

That's a simple insight, yet profound. It explains why in our state and federal governments, low-level solutions are the norm because the political rewards for thinking and acting deeply are just not there.

It also explains why at the federal level, a primary goal is to get the states to generate their own plans and their own solutions. If Washington politicians do not see a clear and present reward for getting involved, they will pass the ball down to the states at every opportunity.

SOCIAL DETERMINANTS OF HEALTH: INSIGHTS FROM CHILMARK RESEARCH'S IT SOLUTIONS TO ENGAGE COMMUNITY RESEARCH REPORT, 2020

Alex Lenox-Miller is a senior analyst with Chilmark Research, a small consulting firm in Boston. Prior to joining Chilmark, Alex was head of analytics for process improvement at Lahey Health, a Massachusetts-based organization that manages hospitals, physicians, and other health services in northeastern Massachusetts. Healthcare is almost literally in Alex's bloodstream.

"My wife is a nurse," Alex tells me. "My mother is a doctor. I found working within the provider system phenomenally Interesting, but very difficult. I'm a change-oriented person. I like fixing things, I like making improvements, making a bunch of small granular improvements that add up to major changes. And that's really hard from within a provider organization. And being able to really push that change from my current position is what I like most."

When it comes to understanding healthcare trends, Alex has among the broadest perspectives and is surely one of the best informed.

And here is one of his most interesting, and most telling, perspectives:

"One of the things that we're seeing really take off now is that some of the biggest pushers of technology aren't providers at all, they're payers and they're employers."

Social Determinants of Health: Insights from Chilmark Research's IT Solutions to Engage Community Research Report, 2020 is just one of many research-based reports from Chilmark that highlight the kind of changes that Alex is referring to.

Here are some of the key takeaways from the report:

- As emphasis on value-based care becomes more prevalent, providers and payers are seeking to address social determinants of health (SDOH) in their patient populations to lower utilization costs.

- To do so, the providers and payers must engage with organizations capable of affecting changes in aspects of patients' lives that traditionally existed outside of the scope of healthcare. Vendors are rising to meet the need by connecting these organizations (called community resources or community partners) to various healthcare organizations so that both may benefit from coordination in service provisioning.

- Integration with community partners remains the main barrier to implementation, given challenges with data governance. Legal and internal engagement issues also slow adoption.

- Providers that wish to address patients' social needs can do so efficiently through referrals to community partners. This is made dramatically easier with community resource engagement solutions.

- The next two years will bring expansion of product capabilities with slow and steady growth in implementation as the market better defines standards for performance. Years three through five will see accelerated adoption and growth.

- The steady march to value-based care (VBC) amplifies interest in solutions that contribute to utilization management strategies.

- Within five years, a public option for insurance will dramatically increase the rate of solutions adoption, culminating in 80 percent adoption in provider locations by 2030.

- Key benefits for taking part in community engagement resource solutions include: the ability to make self-referrals to sources of information and care (for patients); the ability to coordinate care (for providers); and to manage patient relationships more effectively (for community partners).

HOW NEW TECHNOLOGIES GAIN ACCEPTANCE

"One of the things that we're seeing now really take off is that some of the biggest pushers of new technology aren't providers at all," Alex says. "They're payers and they're employers. Those entities are so much more flexible and agile in terms of adoption of technologies—and maybe less clinically driven.

"Provider organizations have been more hesitant to adopt this stuff but there are exceptions. Some of them are a lot more forward-looking than others but by and large, have been really hesitant to adopt a lot of the newer digital health technologies for a variety of reasons. They often fear they lose the ability to control or drive usage by virtue of that change in dynamics and that digital health is forced on providers by new market dynamics when they didn't have a solution in place. They're still scrambling—they don't have unified workflows and they don't have unified technology."

SPEAKING WITH PETER V. LEE, EXECUTIVE DIRECTOR, COVERED CALIFORNIA

There is certainly no shortage of industry pundits and naysayers in healthcare. It seems like everyone can message the problems. There is no shortage of opinion on who are the heroes and villains. Yet, turning that insight and sometimes vitriol into actionable policy that drives benefits has proven to be elusive. After about twelve years in healthcare, I can honestly say I have met very few people like Peter Lee. He may just be a unicorn.

After speaking with Peter for only a few minutes, you realize that he cares deeply for the wellbeing of people not only in his state, but everywhere. Peter is the first Executive Director for California's health benefit exchange, Covered California. Having been confirmed unanimously by the exchange board in 2011, he now oversees the planning, development, ongoing administration and evaluation of Covered California and its efforts to improve the affordability and accessibility of quality healthcare for Californians.

A BIT OF CALIFORNIA HEALTHCARE HISTORY

California's first health benefit exchange was established by the state in September 2010 to support the expansion of coverage enabled by the Affordable Care Act of 2010. As the first state to create a health benefit exchange following the passage of federal healthcare reform, it is charged with creating a new insurance marketplace where individuals and small businesses can purchase competitively priced healthcare plans using federal tax subsidies and credits.

Prior to his current role as executive director of Covered California, Peter served as the deputy director for the Center for Medicare and Medicaid Innovation at the Centers for Medicare and Medicaid Services (CMS) in Washington, D.C. where he led initiatives to identify, test and support new models of care in Medicare and Medicaid, resulting in higher quality care while reducing costs.

Previously, Peter was the director of Delivery System Reform for the Office of Health Reform for the U.S. Department of Health and Human Services, where he coordinated delivery reform efforts for Secretary Kathleen Sebelius and assisted in the preparation of the National Quality Strategy. Before joining the Obama

Administration, he served from 2000-2008 as the CEO and executive director for National Health Policy of the Pacific Business Group on Health (PBGH), one of the leading coalitions of private and public purchasers in the nation. Peter also served from 1995-2000 as the executive director of the Center for Healthcare Rights, a consumer advocacy organization based in Los Angeles, and he was the former director of programs for the National AIDS Network.

Prior to his work in public service, Peter was a practicing attorney in Los Angeles. A native Californian, Peter holds a juris doctorate from the University of Southern California and a B.A. from the University of California, Berkeley.

AN OVERVIEW OF THE MARKETPLACES

Peter observes that before the Affordable Care Act, individuals who did not have employer-based insurance generally faced three major impediments to obtaining healthcare coverage.

The first challenge was affordability. Could they afford coverage? If they couldn't, where could they get financial help? Did employers help to pay for coverage? Peter points out that in that individual market, healthcare consumers received no financial help, no tax write-offs, and no tax benefits.

The second challenge that Peter cites is that then-in-force insurance rules precluded people who needed coverage from getting it. This problem is still present and was noted during the years of the Trump presidency. Donald Trump said that under his "plan," consumers would be protected if they had preexisting conditions. But did that provide coverage for the majority of Americans? No. Peter points out that insurers generally were only able to make money by refusing to provide coverage to people who were already sick. Peter notes, "That was the business model."

The third challenge, according to Peter, was that pre-ACA, healthcare was a kind of "Wild West," with no standards. People generally didn't know what was covered, and what wasn't. They would sign up for coverage and suddenly discover that specific forms of care, like care for mental health, wasn't part of their plan. And often, the types of care that weren't covered were those that led consumers to sign up for coverage in the first place.

How much have those limitations and problems changed?

Peter summarizes, "So the ACA, is almost 10 years ago and has changed how we manage each of those challenges in big waves, even in the employer market. It set standard benefit designs and you're going to get penalized as an employer if you don't provide some sort of minimum coverage. But for the poor people that don't have employer coverage, what about them?

"People say, well, it's one thing to change the rules so that insurers could not turn people away. They had to make sure that everyone's acceptance would be based on factors like risk adjustment. If you were a healthcare plan that somehow managed to break the rules and avoid people with, say, cancer or diabetes, those people would still get money from you as a health plan to help them pay for the care they needed. That level of risk adjustment was huge."

Plus, we have to remember that in the pre-ACA system, similar to today, about half of Americans got coverage through their employers. And that employer coverage was supported by federal tax dollars; that was a tax-free benefit to the employee. So federal money, to the tune of hundreds of billions of dollars? We taxpayers helped pay for that.

Peter points out that the ACA helped more people pay for their coverage by doing two things: First, by expanding Medicaid; and second, by providing tax credits for people who made too much money to be eligible for Medicaid.

"The Supreme Court said, you cannot make every state automatically expand Medicaid, it needs to be an option," Peter tells me. "But with that, 39 states now have expanded Medicaid. You get, in essence, free coverage to go into the Medicaid population. California expanded Medicaid. About three million more Californians got Medicaid coverage, many coming through us. The other thing it did was give advance premium tax credits, giving consumers financial help that is adjusted for their income, thereby helping them buy coverage and get better coverage. So lower income people get more money, higher income people get less money, but still get financial help."

"In California, we've signed up 250,000 people since Covid, more than double what we signed up a year before. We have seen dramatic increases. But that doesn't just happen all by itself. You have Covered California doing marketing outreach to let people know what is available. You've got Medicaid expansion in Texas. You have a federal marketplace. Under the previous administration, Healthcare.gov was not spending a dime on marketing. It doesn't tell you where to go and doesn't have a Medicaid program to expand. If you lose your employer-based coverage in Texas, chances are you are going to be out of luck. Some people may be eligible for the marketplace, tax credits, subsidies—but many won't.

"The main thing the pandemic does is highlight the inconsistencies nationally of when you have states being able to opt in and out of healthcare saying we won't expand Medicaid and will rely on the whim of the federal government to decide to do all our marketing to promote people using the marketplace to buy their healthcare insurance. You're basically allowing people to have their lives not be secured by consistent policies, but at the whim of what states do and inconsistencies of employer-based coverage.

"We have a federal system that allows states to make decisions. Some of the blocking and tackling is the state taking the decision to expand Medicaid. And one of the fascinating stories to me is the ten or fifteen very red states that have acted to expand their Medicaid program. Most recently Missouri—by a state ballot amendment, the voters said, we disagree with our Republican governor and a Republican legislature, expand the damn Medicaid program. Yeah, and they're still a red state."

HOW THIS AFFECTS THE
MAN OR WOMAN IN THE STREET

Let's see how this plays out in different states. (Bear with me, this gets a bit complex.) if you're eligible for Medicaid in California, you can get that. If you make too much money to be eligible for Medicaid in California, that's called MediCal.

In other states, it can play out quite differently. If you lived in Colorado and were making $25,000 a year, you might get $300 a month from federally administered Medicare to help you buy the plan you want. And you would get a selection of different plans you could choose from, based on what's been put on the shelf in the marketplace. If you're not eligible for financial help, you can still pick those plans and those same plans are available through a marketplace or in the individual market at the same exact price.

"So that's the basic structure," Peter explains. "What's different among marketplaces is the extent to which a marketplace negotiates with health plans."

But the way it is all administered is somewhat more distilled and refined in California.

Peter explains, "I think it's clear we are the largest marketplace in the nation except for Healthcare.gov. The other 12 state-based marketplaces in sum have collective enrollment the same as Californians. We are big, but we were formed by the state of California to be an independent entity. Our job at Covered California is to get as many people insured as possible to supplement and complement Medicaid, MediCal in California. But to promote better healthcare, we do everything we can."

CALIFORNIA COMPARED TO NATIONAL TRENDS

Since Covered California opened its doors, premiums nationwide have gone up an average of seven percent or so a year. And over the last two years, they have gone up less than one percent in California.

But for context, let's compare that to what happened in the federal marketplace, where premiums went up at about double the rate in California. That means that people who do not live in California, and who don't get subsidies, have been forced out of healthcare due to rising premiums.

Peter explains that even healthy people are saying, "I can't afford this."

"They've been priced out," Peter explains. "We now have an environment where there are two challenges. Many people that are nominally eligible for the individual market but are not subsidy-eligible in much of the nation are out of luck. They can't afford it.

"But we've also seen that many people, in employer-based coverage, have coverage that isn't affordable for them. Remember what we do as a structure, and I know you're really talking about what do you do if you're not covered by an employer plan?

"According to a new report from the Commonwealth Foundation, 43 percent of adults are inadequately insured. Most have employer coverage, but they've got high deductible plans and the vast majority of employer coverage doesn't do what we do in California, which adjusts our contributions based on your income. Say you make $200,000 or you make $20,000, you pay the same share of a monthly premium. That is cuckoo. It's not fair. It doesn't promote healthcare coverage. And I think one of the things we'll see going forward after the pandemic is a renewed focus on the inequities.

"So how did we succeed? We actually did most of the things that the tools were there for. And we did them pretty well. Our IT work people focused on infrastructure. People have good choices to choose amongst. And we've promoted the heck out of it, so we get a good risk pool and have shown dramatically lower cost."

COVERED CALIFORNIA IN CONTEXT

By population, California equals about six other states combined.

To look at it another way, the population of Vermont is less than 700,000 people. That is one-third of just the Sacramento metropolitan area, which is the fourth largest metropolitan area in California.

California rural areas have increased at a slightly higher rate than the average of the entire state, but not a lot higher. Peter points out that L.A. may have seven health plans to choose from, but 80 percent of the enrollees across the state have three or more plans to choose from.

"I can guarantee you that Vermont, as a percentage of premium, is not going to spend $150 million," Peter summarizes. "We're a big state. But look at it as a percentage of premium. And the things we're doing absolutely can be replicated across the state, across the nation, and generally are."

THE EXTRAS THAT CALIFORNIA HAS ADDED

California has done a number of things that other states haven't. It has created standard benefit designs that differ according to where consumers live.

Peter explains that, depending on location, consumers can have anywhere from two or three to seven health plans to choose from. Yet there are 11 health plans that are offered throughout the state. If you are in L.A. as an example, seven different health plans are available. If you want a Silver-level product, which could be a product with a deductible of $1,500, every one of those Silver products between Blue Cross Health to Kaiser, is identical.

For consumers, that means comparing apples to apples. They're saying, OK, I want this. I want Kaiser versus HealthNet because I like their network of doctors, not because of some benefit design. The other thing California did by having standard designs is that even though the Affordable Care Act says there are 10 essential benefits, and the standard designs are worth something, actuarial value means a Silver plan covers 70 percent of your costs and you pay 30 percent. "That's what a 70 percent Silver plan is," Peter explains.

"But that could mean many different things in terms of what's your deductible. How much do you pay when you see a doctor? For us in California, it's standardized. And for our Silver plan, which is the most common plan people choose, while there's a deductible, the deductible never applies to outpatient care. So you go see your doctor and get first dollar coverage. [Coverage with no deductible – Ed.] You don't have to spend $1,500 before your insurance kicks in. You need an X-ray out of the hospital? First dollar coverage. You need drugs paid for first? And again, every one of our plans does the same thing."

"This is an advantage to living in California—that first-dollar coverage. And it is very humane. Virtually no other states offer anything like that. And the feds don't do that. So what that means is if you're in Denver, Colorado, or in Atlanta, Georgia," Peter clarifies, "and you go to their marketplace and say, 'I want to pick a plan,' you won't just see five carriers competing to offer one of those Silver-level plans. Each of those carriers might have three variations of Silver products. People are confused. They don't know what they're getting. We think it's bad for consumers."

But in California, Peter and his colleagues at Covered California "curate" the plans that people can choose. "'Curate' is exactly the term we use for it," Peter explains. "Curation came in vogue a few years ago. But so, yes, we absolutely curate it. And we do that based on behavioral economics."

In California, many of the people who lost their jobs are low-income service industry workers. Who are the first people to lose their jobs? It's people in retail. People in food service. Many of them didn't have insurance except for MediCal because their employers weren't offering coverage. What we saw, and we're still analyzing this, is that the huge changes in employment didn't reflect huge changes of insurance, because many of these people were already in MediCal. That said, I think that one of the things the pandemic and the recession that followed it highlighted is when you talk about fixing healthcare and it taking a village, the last thing you want in a pandemic is people to be uninsured.

Peter states, "Having people have insurance and healthcare insecurity because they've lost job-based coverage and need to look around is part of the craziness of a system that is such a patchwork. Today, there is not an automatic process that the moment you lose your job-based coverage, you're automatically enrolled in the lowest cost plan through Covered California, and you pay what you can. Rather, you're thrown to the wolves. Now, you're lucky in California, where you've got us as a shepherd, we've curated the market and are keeping the wolves at bay.

"The other thing we do, we look at our vision, our mission statement. We want to have people get the right care at the right time and lower costs. Part of that means we aren't just about giving people an insurance card. We want to make sure once they get enrolled, they get the right care at the right time. We have high expectations of our health plans to make sure that people with diabetes are well cared for. We have a medical director and a physician team looking over the shoulders of our health plans to make sure they are getting the right care at the right time."

A NEW KIND OF INCLUSIVENESS

But one thing is undeniable about the way California manages its healthcare coverage. Insurers are unable to avoid sick people. And they are unable to discriminate according to income and other economic factors.

"We want to get everyone in the door," Peter says. "We have as few barriers as possible."

In support of that inclusiveness, Peter and his team do a phenomenal amount of marketing and promotion.

There is no doubt that Peter and his Covered California team have raised the bar and helped to build a system that can serve as a positive example for every state in the nation. Those accomplishments spring in part from Peter's compassion and belief in helping people.

"Healthcare's gotten better," he summarizes. "That was part of why I left the Obama administration to come to California. We had a state that was ready to say, it's not just a marketplace. We shouldn't just be putting gobbledygook on the shelf and hoping consumers can figure it out. We should be curating a market and holding health plans accountable. And part of curating a market is putting good products on the shelf. But part of it's also doing a lot of marketing, so we get more people in. And over the last seven years, we have demonstrated that it works."

It does indeed work. California has created healthcare's best practice template for marketplaces that other states can emulate with benefit for their residents. In addition to a curated experience, they have also done a stellar job of aggregating subsidies to make healthcare affordable for all Californians. How long will it be before you can choose Medicare as one of the options on Covered CA? Stay tuned. Peter Lee is a man on a mission and that mission includes making sure everyone has total access to quality affordable care.

LET'S HEAR FROM VERMONT

We mentioned Vermont a few pages ago—that state with the population that could practically fit into a corner of Los Angeles. Or, as we like to say back home in Vermont, still more cows than people! Let's explore what is going on there, because when we consider one of the states that has a smaller population than California, we can learn important lessons about how healthcare is being administered in smaller areas with transient residents who often live seasonably in other states.

So, what is similar? Surprisingly, a number of things. For one, a sizeable percentage of the people in the state lack coverage. Another similarity is that the percentage of people who lost their jobs during the pandemic is not all that different. A number of them are undocumented and lack coverage. A number of the people who lost their jobs during the pandemic are front-line workers in retail and food service industries.

Although many of the challenges that these two states are confronting are similar in outline, significant differences have arisen in the way they administer their healthcare programs.

To get an insider's view, I spoke with Kevin Mullin. chair of the Green Mountain Care Board (gmcboard.vermont.gov). Peter directs the board's charge of curbing healthcare cost growth and reforming the way healthcare is provided to Vermonters.

Although it is a rather rough equivalency, let me say that Kevin Mullin is the Peter Lee of Vermont in that both of these executives care deeply about the people who reside in their states, and both have worked hard to provide care that is both high-quality and attainable.

VERMONT IN CONTEXT

In rankings of the states with the healthiest population, Vermont usually comes in the top five. In the year 2019, they were rated number one in the country.

That shows that when it comes to providing health coverage and care for its people, Vermont is clearly doing a lot of things well. But there are issues to confront. In rural areas of the state, you will find populations of people who are obese, who smoke, who have diabetes, who lack access to good nutrition. Yes, even in a state where people are surrounded by farmer's fields and dairy farms, poor diet comes into play same as anywhere else.

But overall, compared to the other states, Vermont's doing a good job. And the people in charge are committed to continuing to do so. According to Kevin, "One of the key areas of focus in our all-payer model agreements is to focus on prevention and wellness.

"We're focusing on the fact that chronic illnesses are really 80 percent of the cost of the system. Because of that, we are focusing on issues like pre-diabetes. When I first took this position, I was invited down to Brattleboro Memorial Hospital, which is in the southeast corner of the state, and they were so proud to show me their new wound treatment center with the hyperbaric chambers and other advanced technologies. And they were going on and on how they were able to treat wounds, so people didn't have to have amputations. But I asked, 'What are you doing with your primary care doctors in the community to start addressing this?'

"When people first start showing signs of pre-diabetes, you can address this problem, so they never get to the stage where they have wounds that you need to treat. And that's really where the big dollar savings can occur if you can get somebody to change their lifestyle early on, change their exercise, change their nutrition habits, that's key.

"As part of the agreement with the federal government, we're focused on three key areas. The biggest is chronic illnesses, but we're also focused on trying to lower deaths from overdose and to lower suicide rates. You would think that a rural area might be immune from substance abuse, but we're not. And we have all the same problems as the rest of the country. We are working on those areas. We're trying to do innovative programs. For example, we started a VeggieVanGo program that gets fresh vegetables in the hands of people in the community that probably wouldn't be able to afford them otherwise. Whether outside of schools or medical clinics, there are bags of fresh vegetables that are ready to go for people. And people are very receptive to it."

ON BEING LITTLE

"Because of our size, we're kind of unique compared to other states," Kevin says, "so we don't have for-profits competing with one another here. We don't even have multiple hospitals in any health service area competing with each other.

"It is very small, which is both a blessing and a curse. Because of our size, we're often able to convince the federal government to allow us to try things, to see if they work. And hence, right now, we're under an agreement with the federal government on an all-payer model agreement. And those are the type of things that our small size helps us to accomplish.

"We have very limited provider competition and because of that, we believe that intense regulation has to occur because something has to be a moderating force. There is no competition for pricing or anything like that. We have to do that through regulation. We are also always trying to balance achieving efficiencies through economies of scale with issues like transportation because of our rural nature.

"Technologies are an example of the issues we had to address that were highlighted by Covid-19. We covered about three years of forward progress on telehealth in about three weeks, out of necessity. One of the drawbacks is that there are areas of the state that have very limited access to broadband. So those are the kinds of deficiencies that we're trying to correct. The state is now trying to argue the use of some of the federal coronavirus relief funds be used for improving our technological infrastructure."

THE COMMERCIAL HEALTH COVERAGE MARKET IN VERMONT

Vermont's healthcare landscape is not overcrowded—there are Blue Cross, MVP, Aetna and Cigna.

But this quickly gets complex—Aetna and Cigna are not selling products on Vermont's healthcare exchange.

"Our exchange is different from a lot of others," Kevin explains, "in that we have a combined exchange. Our exchange covers individuals and small groups. So that is something that is different from a lot of other states. We've struggled with workforce, but I think all states have struggled with it too. We genuinely don't know what will happen.

"We've been working pretty hard in Vermont to expand coverage, access and affordability, because we don't have the competition that would typically bring down pricing. In 2011, I was put in charge of the Green Mountain Care Board, and we have some pretty strong levers. For example, we determine what the growth rate will be for a hospital—that's the growth in their net patient revenue and fixed perspective payments. They can't just add on utilization and grow their way into expansion. In addition to that, we also have to approve any change of charges which again gets carried forward on to reimbursement rates from the carriers. We have some pretty heavy levers here in Vermont to deal with the fact that we don't have a competitive market. It seems to be working, but time will tell.

"We were way ahead of the Affordable Care Act and tried to expand that coverage in Vermont. For example, in 2006, we created an insurance program called Catamount Health, which has since gone by the wayside when we started the Vermont Health Exchange.

"But basically, what Catamount did was it provided state subsidies for employer-sponsored insurance, and we reduced our own insurance rate that way."

HOW MANY CONSUMERS
IN VERMONT HAVE COVERAGE?

According to Kevin, three percent of Vermonters are currently uninsured. Participation is measured using the Vermont Household Data Survey, which is a phone survey that polls Vermonters about their coverage.

Respondents are asked a lot of questions about whether they have coverage, and what kind of coverage they do have. Kevin has been surprised to learn that participation across the state has remained fairly constant, at about three percent, for the last two years, which included one year pre-Covid, and one during the first year of the pandemic.

Kevin says, "I thought there would have been an uptick once the penalty for not having insurance was removed. But that hasn't occurred yet. I still worry about that. What is a bigger problem, though, is the underinsured, because we have a larger segment of the population going towards high deductible plans? And that has just as much concern for us as the uninsured rate."

WHY COMPETITION ISN'T ALWAYS
GOOD IN A SMALL STATE LIKE VERMONT

It's a valid assumption that where healthcare coverage is concerned, competition is a force that increases both quality and affordability. But in a closed system like Vermont, other considerations come into play.

Kevin points out that competition doesn't necessarily lead to better outcomes. He points out that the goal is to have "the right care, at the right time, in the right setting."

"Let's consider heart surgery," he says. "We don't want all 14 community hospitals in Vermont to be doing that. For one thing, there's a lot of research that shows if you don't do something often enough, you don't get the quality and the results that you want. We want the right setting in the community, but if you need that more comprehensive care, we want you to go to a tertiary medical center like the University of Vermont or in our case, a lot of care, especially on the eastern side of the state, goes to Dartmouth."

HOW VERMONT SERVED ITS
CITIZENS DURING THE COVID-19 PANDEMIC

Because Vermont has its own state healthcare exchange that has the goal of meeting the needs of Vermonters, it was able to flexibly open its enrollment period and make it easy for people who lost their jobs to get on the exchange.

"It was a very good thing for our state that we have that flexibility, and we have that control," Kevin says, "I will say that it wasn't without problems. And when the exchange was first set up, it was somewhat of a disaster as the technology was not really up for the challenges. But slowly but steadily, that has come under control.

But for a while, it was very trying on consumers in Vermont who were trying to get that product."

SO, WHAT IS HAPPENING AT THE STATE LEVEL IN HEALTHCARE ACROSS AMERICA?

There is no one answer to that question. There are 50, because there are 50 states. Actually, there are more than 50 answers, because the District of Columbia and all the U.S. territories have different approaches.

The smarter people we have working on the issues we have explored here, the better chances of aligning policy, public and private offerings so people can get and stay healthy. That is encouraging.

Whether you live in a large state like California or a smaller state like Vermont, the challenge of providing residents with total access to quality affordable care is the mission. If you get a sense that Californians and Vermonters have a leg up, you are probably right. We need more people like Peter Lee and Kevin Mullin who eat, breathe and sleep this stuff. While many in healthcare simply go through the motions, these men won't rest until they have significantly moved the needle and improved healthcare in their home states. I thoroughly expect Medicare will soon be a choice you can make in our exchanges and will not be surprised if California and Vermont are leading that charge. We all deserve totally unencumbered access to healthcare, but we can't take our eyes off the equally important targets of quality and cost.

CHAPTER SEVEN
LIFE HACKS

We have covered a lot of ground in the last six chapters. But you have probably noted that we have surveyed it from a fairly elevated perspective, viewing the "big picture" trends, laws, and predictions.

Let's take our virtual helicopter down closer to the ground level and ask a more immediate question:

If you're enjoying the results of all these "It Takes a Village" trends, what technologies are you using, and what are they doing for you?

WHAT NEW DIGITAL TOOLS HAVE LANDED IN YOUR DIGITAL TOOLBOX IN THE LAST TWO YEARS?

The two years since I wrote *The Digital Healthcare Revolution* are a very short period of time. But thanks to the quickening pace of innovation and change, at least a decade's worth of innovation has taken place in that time, maybe even more. Some of that acceleration is due to the Covid-19 pandemic and the demands it placed on healthcare.

Hundreds, if not thousands, of new apps have landed on our phones. Do you want to manage your body mass index, remember to engage in a guided meditation, listen to white noise so you can sleep better, or keep track of your ovulation cycle or sperm count (yes, there are apps for that) and have a baby sooner? You can do all those things, and more, because you have landed in a digital promised land.

But there is more to innovation than just a growing number of apps. Here are some of the larger trends that I see at work.

There is increasing integration of a wider range of health-related functions. Two years ago, we were predicting a time when a customer who was in the office of her primary care provider could immediately and seamlessly schedule a visit with a specialist, schedule tests, have a prescription filled at her pharmacy, and have everything approved by her health insurance plan. And two years later, that kind of integration is already here. All the different segments of the care experience are sliding together like the cylinders of a telescope fitting into each other.

Boundaries of other kinds are evaporating too. If you got diagnosed with, say, type 2 diabetes two years ago, your primary care physician sent you to a specialist who in turn sent you to a nutritionist who printed out a list of foods that you folded up and took to a food store. Now those boundaries are vanishing, and the entire care experience is becoming much more frictionless. It could just be that the time is here when you can be diagnosed with type 2 when you are in a pharmacy like a Walgreens or a CVS, where you can also visit with a nutritionist. From there, without even going outside the building, you will walk into a food store where a shopper will have a basket full of the foods you need to start your new diet from a list you developed while with your nutritionist. If you do not already belong to a gym, that will be a part of the sign-up process as well. You won't have to contact your health insurance plan to get approvals or submit requests for payment. It will all happen as one process, neatly monitored on your phone and integrated with all your benefits.

You feel better, eat better, exercise more, and simply *live* better than ever before. Plus, you can expect to keep living a lot longer, healthier life. I know plenty of people who have hit age 70 while still feeling as youthful and energetic as they did half a century ago. I know people who are vibrant and energized at age 80, or even 90 and sometimes beyond. These are the benefits that have resulted from the convergence of a number of trends, including better care, a greater emphasis on exercise and nutrition, and even the normalization of certain conditions like depression. Things are getting better—a lot better. What an exciting time this is to be alive.

Yes, we are landing firmly on the ground. And now that we are there, let's meet our guides—bright, futuristic company leaders—who will explain what they are doing for consumers of healthcare. Maybe one of their customers is . . . you?

HOW HAS THE MARKETPLACE CHANGED IN THE LAST TWO YEARS?

In my last book *The Digital Health Revolution*, I included this list of companies that were making fitness monitors:

- Adidas
- Charge
- Fitbit
- Flex
- Fossil
- Garmin
- Huawei
- Jawbone
- Kua
- Life Trak
- Mio
- Misfit
- Moov

- Polar
- Samsung
- TomTom
- Under Armour
- Withings
- Xiaomi

Today, the landscape is expanding quickly, and includes a variety of wearable devices that do a lot more than monitor your exercise and fitness. Here's a quick list of companies that are moving into the wearable technology marketplace, most with devices and technologies that measure a variety of health factors that go well beyond fitness and exercise. Note too that the companies that are included on both the list above and the list below have generally expanded from offering wearables that monitored only exercise and are now offering devices that monitor a larger selection of health indicators.

Some of the new entrants and important players are:

- Apple
- Facebook
- Fitbit
- Garmin
- Google
- HTC
- Huawei
- Lumen
- Microsoft
- Oura
- Qualcomm
- Samsung
- Sony
- Vusix
- Xiaomi

BRINGING AI TO WELLNESS, BEHAVIORAL HEALTH, AND MEDICAL CARE DELIVERY: TALKING WITH DR. MURRAY ZUCKER, CORPORATE MEDICAL OFFICER OF HAPPIFY HEALTH

The future of technology in healthcare can be as unlimited as our imaginations. Tech innovation has already started ushering in positive, significant changes. For instance, we just witnessed the rapid adoption of telemedicine during the pandemic. And given the mental health crisis that pre-existed the pandemic and has become much worse since, imagine a world where behavioral health treatment, enhanced by AI, can reach more people in an efficient and effective manner with data to prove progress. Well, the future is here and about to get even better.

Here's something to consider—what if the treatment you're receiving on your smartphone, laptop, or computer is not with a human, but driven by proven digitized therapeutic programs with AI to personalize your experience and improve outcomes and engagement?

Think of the rapid advances that once seemed impossible a short while ago and are now taken for granted by us—Siri and Alexa answering our questions, finding things, and adjusting our home environment. In addition to present AI enhancement, soon embedded voice recognition, natural language processing, data from wearables, and integrated data from smartphones—which are proxies of physiologic markers of one's mental and physical status—will allow much more accurate and individualized treatment. This can be an adjunct to the usual treatment or may be available for the overwhelming number of people who don't access treatment.

One company leading this field is Happify Health (Happify Health.com) which is delivering an expanding range of care. Happify is a global software-enabled healthcare platform company improving behavioral health, physical health, and wellbeing and offering digital therapeutics, prescribed digital therapeutics (it's Ensemble product soon to be released as a pilot), therapeutics with pharma partners, social media platforms for specific disease-related communities, and a platform for integrating benefits and modernizing patient navigation and experience for health plans and employers.

According to Dr. Murray Zucker, Happify's corporate medical officer, Happify is already able to deliver the following AI enabled functions:

- **Treatment using an AI assisted coach called 'Anna,' a patented technology which can determine and adjust to the emotions, moods, and needs of the user and can store responses and data to continually improve the understanding of the user (of course remaining cybersecure and HIPPA compliant).** So if someone is angry or stressed out, the program picks that up and alters the course to help the person immediately deal with the situation.

- **Treatment is in 10 languages and culturally sensitive –** so it's not just a translation. This allows for Happify to be used in many countries, by over 20 million covered lives, many Fortune 500 companies, and some of the biggest health plans in the U.S.

- **The treatments embedded in the app are science-based, validated, and proven effective in the digital format and based on cognitive behavioral therapy (CBT), mindfulness, positive psychology, and other disciplines.** And the engagement rates are the best in the field and are long-lasting.

- **As Happify succeeds, it enables greater access to care, more effective and efficient care, more consistent care, and data to prove it and give feedback to the user, employer, health plan, or pharma customer.**

How has Happify put all this together? I recently sat down for a chat with Dr. Murray Zucker to find out more. As a psychiatrist with a background in academia, large group practice, and health plan clinical leadership, he brings expertise in medical behavioral integration, patient engagement and adherence, health behavior change and new technologies in diagnosis and treatment. Previously, he was senior medical director at Optum Behavioral Health for New Product and Innovation. He graduated University of Pennsylvania, went on to the medical school at University of Rochester, spent two years running a medical clinic on a southwest Indian reservation, and did his psychiatric residency at UCLA where he remained on faculty.

As a media spokesman for mental health, you may have seen him on *The Today Show, Good Morning America, 20/20,* and CNN.

HOW DOES HAPPIFY HEALTH "HELP PEOPLE, ONE PERSON AT A TIME"?

Happify is having a big impact and lives up to its tag line: "helping people, one person at a time." Murray explains, "We take proven, science-based therapeutics, digitize them, wrap them in an engaging interface, and get impressive improvement in stress, anxiety, depression, and resilience as measured by our outcome studies. In this field, you can't afford to take short cuts, and at Happify, we have an entire division dedicated to outcome studies, randomized controlled trials (RTC's), and Health economic and outcomes research (HEOR)." The AI engine in the background learns more and more about the user and personalizes the program while data is analyzed to inform as to progress and trends.

The founders of Happify, Ofer Leidner and Tomer ben-Kiki, were previously successful in the gaming industry, and afterwards they decided to take the lessons learned about gamification, engagement and adherence and apply them to improve health-care. And the result is far superior engagement and lasting continuation with the platform because the apps are enjoyable, interesting, compelling, and useful.

Presently, many of Happify's products have over 3,000 activities and games to choose from, over 65 tracks or mini-programs, and 300 guided meditations as well as daily infographics, and individualized recommendations. Users note their thoughts, monitor activity, join group support, share experiences, and watch their progress.

HELP WHEN PEOPLE NEED IT

One immediate benefit of digital therapy is that it's available to users 24/7–at their time, at their need, at their location. "It isn't like going to a therapist's office once a week and having no idea of the consistency or proficiency of that therapist," Murray says. "Everybody is getting a different version of CBT that way. But with our digital therapeutic you're getting a validated, consistent, and measurable product and you can actually look at outcomes."

IMPORTANT APPLICATIONS OF DATA

Murray goes on to say: "When a health plan or employer provides Happify Health to its members or employees, the individual gets feedback, the therapist gets feedback, and the health plans and employers get population-based feedback that show both improvement and value.

We're fortunate that with digital therapeutics we can reach more people, anywhere, at scale that is affordable, effective, and efficient. And by addressing the stress, anxiety, and depression frequently accompanying many chronic medical illnesses, we can improve quality of life, physical health, and lower healthcare costs."

WHERE HAPPIFY HEALTH IS GOING

As the Covid-19 pandemic winds down, studies and surveys show there has been a massive increase in mental health problems—burnout, anxiety, depression, substance use, eating disorders, child, spouse, and elder abuse, PTSD and worsening for those with chronic mental illness. That's not to mention whatever long lasting mental effects having had the virus may show. Murray adds, "When you look at certain populations—the elderly, teens—the numbers are startling. One survey showed a 25 percent increase in teen suicidality—a five-time increase! The elderly are vulnerable because of loneliness and isolation and perhaps lack of resources. Other vulnerable populations have showed higher than expected rates of infection and mortality. Hopefully, the ever-increasing power of AI and the digital experience can help address these issues as well."

According to Murray, "We have two pandemics—the Covid pandemic and the mental health pandemic. The current manpower in the mental health field is just not capable of handling the need. This is another case for the digital approach to mental and physical health."

Murray points out that "severe depression, for example, will affect people physiologically for years to come. So, for example, if you look at two diabetic patients—one with co-existing depression (about 50 percent have this)—guess what? The depressed diabetic needs more insulin, has more hospitalizations for medical problems, more foot infections and other complications. if you can reduce the anxiety and/or depression in the chronically medically ill, you really improve quality of life and decrease medical expenditure. Digital therapeutics makes this more likely."

I think that anyone who perceives technology as remote, distant, and non-caring would do well to think about the views that Murray shared. When the people behind the technology are not only scientists and clinicians but also dedicated to doing good and helping people, that technology becomes a powerful vehicle for improving healthcare and the "health of one person at a time."

MEET THE LUMEN METABOLISM TRACKER

Truthfully, I could have decided to profile many of the devices I listed above. But I chose to dig in and describe the Lumen Metabolism Tracker for you, because its story is in many ways similar to the story of many other devices, and its development is emblematic of one of the bigger trends—it started essentially as a fitness tracker but evolved to deliver a wider understanding of the wearer's health.

The story of the birth of the Lumen company falls right in line with the stories of other companies we have explored earlier in this book. Like many of those companies, Lumen was born when a few engaged entrepreneurs had a personal epiphany and journey that led them to focus on fitness, wellness and health. And their companies, and the products they developed and brought to market, resulted.

In Lumen's case, two young Israeli women were the impetus. They are twins Michal and Merav Mor, both of whom have earned advanced degrees in physiology. When they were training for an Ironman about five years ago, they started to tinker with a device they could use to measure the CO_2 in their breath.

BILLED AS THE FIRST DEVICE
TO "HACK YOUR METABOLISM"

That experience was the genesis of the Lumen Metabolism Tracker, a very attractive small device that Lumen now sells. It looks like a small, phone-sized device that has a hole on one end that the user breathes into. The data that is collected is immediately transferred to a phone app. The Metabolism Tracker is currently priced at about $350.

BEYOND CO_2

Michal and Merav, as you might have predicted, soon began to do more with their tracker than simply provide users with data about the CO_2 levels in their bloodstreams. The Mor twins were soon envisioning and offering insights from their tracker that allow users to engage in a number of activities that impact their health.

People who use the Lunen Tracker and its app are now:

- Adjusting their exercise routines and enjoying better results

- Adjusting their diet to release more energy from the foods they eat

- Analyzing and better understanding their metabolism

- Receiving a "daily plan" from the app with guidance on sleep, diet, and exercise

- Establishing "metabolic flexibility," which they define as the ability to metabolize fats and carbohydrates optimally

- Getting comprehensive meal plans

THEY CALL THIS A "HACK," BUT I AM NOT SO SURE

I know the term "hack" is very popular today. To me, it implies a dramatically simplified process that results from taking a complicated process and reducing it to a minimalized activity that takes only a minute or two.

Lumen offers a range of actionable information that empowers users to take control of complex processes and activities. It is a very useful tool that offers benefits to people who are committed to achieving better health and who recognize that what they eat plays an important role.

MEET HARPREET SINGH RAI, CEO OF OURA

Harpreet Singh Rai, a true renaissance man in the world of healthcare, studied electrical engineering at the University of Michigan. He launched his business career with Morgan Stanley's merger and acquisitions group, then went on to lead the technology, media, and telecom portfolio for nine years at Eminence Capital.

Today, Harpreet is Chief Executive Officer of Oura, as well as a member of its board. And like other entrepreneurs we have met in this book, Harpreet is involved in healthcare because he has a mission to improve health and wellbeing. Under his leadership, Oura has grown to a team of over 150 employees and has launched its new generation 2 ring, shipping over 300,000 units to 98 different countries. He is responsible for Oura's vision and strategy and guides decisions that ensure the organization's financial health.

WHAT IS AN OURA SLEEP RING?

According to Harpreet, "It's kind of like a Fitbit that you wear on your finger instead of on your wrist only we track different things."

Both a Fitbit and an Oura ring contain sensors, but they are completely different devices with different purposes and missions. I have been a daily wearer of an Oura Sleep Ring for about a year now.

Oura combines advanced sensor technology and a minimal design with an easy-to-use mobile app to deliver precise, personalized health insights straight from your body. Harpreet and the scientists behind the ring have found that the quality and quantity of data that is transmitted through your finger is greater than that transmitted by your wrist.

Day and night, Oura helps you track what the company describes as three simple scores: Readiness, Sleep, and Activity. While you're awake, Oura captures data that reflects your activity and movement. When you're sleeping, Oura captures meaningful data as nighttime is the best opportunity to get an accurate read on your overall health as your body is in a more constant state.

During the day, Oura measures:
- Activity levels
- Calories
- Steps
- Inactive times
- Naps

While you're sleeping, Oura measures:
- Resting heart rate
- Heart rate variability (HRV)
- Respiratory rate
- Body temperature
- Light, deep and REM sleep

- Nighttime movement
- Sleep timing and quality

What benefits have I gotten from wearing an Oura Sleep Ring and using the Oura app? Better sleep is one thing. And as we all know, better sleep translates into an increased feeling of well-being, enhanced energy, and greater mental acuity—and better health too, as indicated by a number of measures. I have experienced all those benefits, and almost certainly more.

TO BENEFIT FROM WEARABLES, PEOPLE HAVE TO ACTUALLY WEAR THEM

Harpreet observes that to create an effective wearable device, it needs to balance accuracy with convenience.

He notes that a device that users wear on their heads could collect an awful lot of useful data, but would people do that? Almost certainly not. Ultimately, Harpreet notes, a wearable device is only valuable if it is actually collecting data. Convenience really matters.

That is very insightful thinking, and it helps explain why Harpreet and his team decided to design a ring. First of all, the Oura Sleep Ring comes in a variety of different finishes and very attractive styles. People wear rings already, so the Oura Ring fits right into something they are already doing.

Harpreet notes that when they are going to bed at night, most people take off their wristwatches. But most of them do not take off their rings. So the Oura Sleep Ring is easy for people to accept and integrate into their daily routines.

WHY YOUR FINGER IS
A GREAT MONITORING LOCATION

"As you know, when people with diabetes are testing their blood glucose, they prick their fingers not their arm or wrist. The blood is close to the surface. With a ring, it's easy to penetrate that deep and get an optical signal. And if you look at it from an electrical engineering perspective, the signal strength here from an optical sense, from your pulse signal is about two thirds of magnitude stronger than most anywhere else on your body. It's stronger for the average person."

Harpreet says that the ring provides "100 times better data" than could be obtained in most other locations on the body. He says that his ring is able to monitor 250 hertz of data, 250 times a second, while most other wearables in workout mode can monitor only between 10 and 50 hertz.

A lot of technology is packed into an Oura Sleep Ring. All the data is monitored and collected, and instantly available on the Oura app on your phone. But part of the magic is that Oura doesn't only serve up data, it interprets it and tells you how ready you are to perform via a Readiness score. Plus, when you wear the ring, you can access a two-week view of your sleep patterns, heart rate changes, average body temperature, and more. No doubt about it, the ring does much more than report on sleep patterns.

INCREASED AWARENESS

I am in my 60s. I work out probably five times a week. I like to track everything. I'm really into all these life hacking things.

After about a month of using the Oura Sleep Ring, I realized that there are certain days when my body doesn't respond as well as it does on other days. I can't seem to get it out of second gear and interestingly enough, I'm finding that those same days correspond with those when I have a low Oura Readiness Score.

I know the point I am about to make is subtle. But the underlying message, I believe, is that it isn't enough to just use a wearable device to collect data. Further, it isn't enough to make sure the data is accurate. What adds value to the process is what you do with the data, and how you interpret it. Oura is making my personal health data actionable, and I am gaining an immediate benefit.

Harpreet gets this and applies a philosophical solution.

"I can track my heart rate every second but how do I benefit?" he says. "That is why we focus on sleep. You can take corrective measures and do something when the data is trending in the wrong direction. The wearable space started off as step trackers and then, morphed into activity trackers. But we believe that sleep is really the foundation of your health. If you look at it from the big point of view, you ask, if you deprive a human of something, how bad does life get? Think about it. If you deprive someone of food, water, sleep, air, what happens? If you deprive a human being of physical activity, they can live for a long time. Basically, you might even be fine. You will lose muscle mass and we don't challenge the notion that exercise is good, but you don't immediately die or become sick if you stop exercising. If you deprive someone of food, that person can last several weeks. Fasting is a real thing. And then if you deprive someone of water, you're probably looking at three to four days before you expire.

"But if you actually take away sleep, and most people don't know this, you could die in a couple of days. Your body will force you to sleep. You'll fall asleep at your desk. You start to lose bodily function. And if you look at sort of the science, the human brain develops while people are sleeping. It's a process of repair and recovery. We know basically all your muscle repair, all your muscle tissue, all your natural growth hormone or most of your testosterone is all released in your sleep. And created in your sleep.

"Research is coming out that shows that if you are deprived of deep sleep, which is linked with the early onset of Alzheimer's. Natural killer T cells that fight off cancer are made when you sleep. So is collagen, which repairs your skin. Because of this, as we conceptualized the Oura Ring, we focused on sleep. It's the foundation of health. Literally, the fountain of youth. But half the people in the U.S. are getting fewer than six hours of sleep a night."

A MINDSET THAT IS RELATED TO RECOVERY AND WELLNESS

It is interesting to note that most people associate wearables with intense levels of exercise and training. If you wear a device that tracks your activity, that somehow implies that you are supposed to be training all the time.

Yet Harpreet mentioned to me the fact that physiologically and metabolically, elite and ultra-fit athletes are quite different from the rest of us—even from those of us who exercise regularly.

For people in that second category (fit people who are not elite athletes), a wearable device can be the catalyst for recovery and healing, which is quite different from being a catalyst to engage in intense training.

And that is where Harpreet and his company's Oura Sleep Ring excel.

CHAPTER EIGHT
THE FUTURE OF HEALTHCARE

So, where is healthcare headed?

If you are like me, some of the most pressing questions are in the following areas:

Telehealth – Is it here to stay, or only a phase? Will it evolve into a virtual care concept that everyone embraces or was it really just driven by a fear of coming in to see your doctor because of the pandemic?

Integration – As you have seen, most of the "moving parts" in the healthcare experience (primary provider care, specialist care, insurance coverage, the delivery of drugs and prescriptions) are folding into becoming unified, seamless processes. I expect that process of reducing friction while better connecting us will continue.

Convenience at the retail level – As you have seen, retail pharmacies are delivering nutritional and other forms of counseling in their locations, plus they are combining that with grocery stores and meal delivery. Retail is blurring the lines and bringing healthcare closer to us in our own neighborhoods. I expect that these trends will continue and expand.

Speed – Gone are the days when you visited your primary care provider, who sent you for tests, visits with specialists, and called your prescriptions to your pharmacy. Now those steps are being completed in just one step. Seamless and integrated is the new normal. Providers not offering this are at risk of losing patients to other providers who can leverage technology to meet people where they are.

The expanding use of smartphones and apps – We have seen a huge explosion and cultural shift over these last ten years. Will it continue?

Let's hear from some of the most forward-thinking visionaries I know in healthcare.

CONSTANCE SJOQUIST, HEALTH TRANSFORMATION ANALYST

Constance Sjoquist is one of the preeminent thought leaders in the health industry today. For more than 25 years, she has guided companies that have been transforming health through disruptive technologies and forward-thinking business strategies to meet the ever-changing landscape of health and technology.

Most recently, Constance was Chief Transformation Officer at HLTH, where she helped create the largest and most important new conference for healthcare innovation. As one of the primary architects in shaping the voice and creating the agenda for a new conversation on how to improve health, Constance leveraged her cross-industry insights into a robust platform for market disruption and industry transformation. During her tenure, HLTH grew from just a concept to one of the leading industry events with over 7,500 senior leaders spanning every corner of health—payers, providers, pharma, employers, policy makers, investors, startups, suppliers, retailers, analysts, and associations—and focused on creating the future of health.

Prior to joining HLTH, Constance was a healthcare research director at Gartner, where she covered digital platforms, health exchanges, consumer personalization and engagement, and payment integrity and fraud, waste, and abuse (FWA) solutions. Prior to joining Gartner, she held senior roles at Optum,

United Healthcare, Blue Cross and Blue Shield of Minnesota, and EngagePoint. She is a member of the Think-X board of advisors.

FROM TELEPHONE TO VIRTUAL CARE

Back in the EAP [Employee Assistance Program] days, employees were given a number by their employer to call if they needed any help, not just with their health, but with what could be called the determinants of health—with finances, marriage, and legal issues, having a kid on drugs, whatever it might have been, even mental health.

"The phone was the way you interacted," Constance says. "There was no EAP clinic or office. All those services came together through the phone. Now we have coaching, telehealth, and other opportunities. So that's going to happen over the phone and that's going to happen if we're fortunate enough to have good Wi-Fi and through Zoom-type meetings.

"And then you had the early days of, let's call it, virtual care. I'm talking about 2008 and 2009, when it got bundled with other benefits. It was really a convenience to begin with. An employee would have a kid with an earache, and it was impossible to drive to a clinic and still get to work on time. Whether parents needed to get a problem dealt with regarding their own health, or their children's, it was that convenience. And now we are in the time of Covid, and we've learned how to better interact with patients virtually.

"Telehealth providers are asking, how good a quality image do I have? Can I capture the right information in this Zoom-type experience? What things can't I capture? I probably can't capture a scope going down your throat. We have learned in the interim what services work well in a virtual world and where we still have growth opportunities for technical advancements. We are in a place where we have no Plan B for how we're going to help that toddler with the earache now. That toddler cannot sit in a waiting room. Thanks to Covid, all this stuff kind of got thrown up in the air right at the same time, but we can use telehealth as an option. The problem is there are all these gaps. What's reimbursable? There are a lot of things that came up from a compliance standpoint, a cost structure standpoint, and a technical/logistical standpoint that the industry is trying to solve very quickly, because if they can't get it right in a pandemic, then when will they?"

CONSTANCE ON THE CHANGING ROLE OF DATA AND DATA INTEGRATION

Constance believes that thanks to improvements we have made to accessing our patient data, we now know a lot more about our care experiences. As our care providers pull information from us and from our diagnostic and other experiences, we will simply know much more about our own health and our conditions and our care too. A more informed patient is a patient more likely to make progress toward getting better.

Constance uses an analogy to explain this trend:

"As an example," she says, "I just mapped a bike ride for friends and family. When I signed up with the app, it asked me my age, my location, my gender. And it also asked me if I wanted to add my wearable devices, and it listed some that I can choose from.

"You may have health-related data we can track from your rides, like your heart rate, whether you are going up or down a hill, whether your heart is going into the red zone. You can almost literally do what we used to do as athletes when we went into the clinic to get stress tested. You can literally use your Map My Ride app, made by Under Armour, which is now into remote detection wearables. And then Map My Ride will ask whether I want to share my information to get a more complete picture of my health. They are helping me track my daily activities so I can better appreciate how everyday life-style choices all add up and affect my overall health.

"Now, do I want Under Armour to be diagnosing my health? Thanks to the app, I now have access to all kinds of information I can decide whether or not to share back to the healthcare system."

"If Map My Ride isn't on the fringe of healthcare, I don't know what is," she says. "My doctor doesn't prescribe it; he doesn't know that I have it. It's not on my health record, but it has intelligence that can be leveraged through partnerships."

ON THE CHANGING ROLE OF PREVENTATIVE DATA

Map My Ride is not collecting this data because they want to be able to say, "You should go to your doctor." They are doing it so they can measure how you are getting healthier.

But Constance has noticed that as a result of using such applications, developing an appreciation for what makes you sick is kicking in. How you develop certain conditions is being discovered. Mind you, this is even more than in the classic seven-minute appointment you typically get with your primary care provider.

She explains, "If I have an arrhythmic heart rate that I don't know about, if I have blood sugar dropping that I don't know about, if I'm hypoglycemic and I don't know it, devices are going to pick up that stuff and tell me that before I even need to go in and see my doctor. It is now becoming sick awareness, health management and not just necessarily health and wealth and fitness, which is where the solutions have been in the past.

"The next phase is going to be the autonomous detection and alerting to health issues. We used to think that meant robots. But it turns out, it is actually just devices picking up intelligence. And making sense of it, to literally better connect us to our healthcare stakeholders who give out clinical advice."

CONSTANCE ON THE DIGITAL DIVIDE

Is all this technology just furthering the gap between those that can afford to see their doctors and access care in other ways, and those who can't? For some people in certain areas of the country, smartphone devices are like a lifeline. People can search, study, get prescriptions, get virtual doctor visits. This has become even more important in the time of Covid because it was harder to travel.

But here is an interesting cultural observation from Constance:

"Did you know that smartphone use is higher in the Hispanic communities than it is in white communities? Many have leap-frogged from the laptop era and moved directly to smartphones. This is going to bring a lot of the solutions to those who are less ingrained in the systems of care.

"I still think the privileged will go to the better clinics and get care. They will still go to the Mayo Clinic instead of using tools on their smartphones, because that is behavior they have adopted. I also think the government still needs to keep everybody on their toes. You don't want private entities deciding what's allowable and what people share."

ON THE ECOSYSTEM OF HEALTHCARE

"Noom is a very interesting company," Constance says. "I'm a bit of a skeptic at heart. I'm old enough to have seen things rise and fall. But when it comes to something like Noom that tracks your shopping, your food choices, what's in your food cart at the store, what's in your refrigerator, it has the opportunity to do what we want it to in other areas.

"One, the food pyramid. We've all found out that wheat and carbohydrates shouldn't be the foundation of our nutritional choices. And then you see all this stuff changing. Every six months, you should or shouldn't do certain things. And when people in large numbers are using these apps and systems and their data is being collected, you now have a body of data. You've given pop health back to the population.

"Through devices that are helping people make decisions, you are giving a lot of information back. Blood test kits are another example. You're giving a lot of information about your family traits, your genomic traits, your community traits (spreading of disease, for example)."

WHAT COMPANIES WILL FAIL?

There is no doubt that a number of companies and technologies will fall by the wayside. They are the ones that are not being helpful or accurate. The ones that really continue to succeed are those that can up the ante around accuracy, around relevance, and around useful outcomes.

Constance summarizes, "If we can turn the percentages to our advantage for losing weight, for not becoming diabetic, for dealing with our mental health, I'll invest in that stuff. If even a few people say, 'This app changed my life.' You have to get out of the obesity bucket and into the lifestyle bucket. And that's a much different approach.

"We have to stop offering carrots and sticks and get to real solutions. Let's say I lost 50 pounds, but in my head, I still think, 'I'm an overweight person.' That problem is always knocking at my door. If I don't constantly keep on this thing, it's going to catch up with me."

STILL MORE VISIONS OF THE FUTURE

We have been talking about making healthcare more of a consumer experience now for about eight to ten years. Yet shopping for your benefits plan is easily one of the most daunting challenges that consumers face.

How can we make that process simpler?

"We need to put ourselves in the shoes of the individual who doesn't have health coverage and needs to figure out how to get it," she says. "For most of us, our first experience in getting our own health plan—separate from one that our parents had us on—was through an employer or we had to go off on our own and look for a non-employer family or individual plan through an agent who showed up in our living room with packets of information to sort through.

"Either way, we were sent a snail mail package or an email message that pointed us to a website or we gathered employees into a meeting space to sift through plan designs, prices, and all kinds of industry jargon like 'out-of-pocket,' 'deductible,' 'in-network,' or 'out-of-network.' In contrast, today, most plans are pretty intuitive and allow customers to adjust according to their preferences and usage. Consumers have become e-commerce centric, and they want their services delivered in an engaging and intuitive manner. Super easy. Super obvious.

"This type of convenience and personalization provides consumers with choices that meet their needs, that they can understand, and, in the end, creates tremendous loyalty because consumers feel their interests are recognized and their demands are met. Just the opposite is true when it comes to purchasing health coverage. Besides being incredibly confusing and only getting one chance each year to choose a plan, there's little guidance available during the process. And if you are looking for a specific type of insurance—say Medicare or a Qualified Health Plan (QHP) that allows you to receive subsidized coverage through a state or federal marketplace—you'll likely need to go to separate websites, all with unique configurations, jargon, and paths to enrollment. Seriously, even some of us within the health industry are challenged to complete the process in one shot and without lingering doubts regarding our selections."

ON DEMOGRAPHIC DIFFERENCES

Does Constance see significant behavioral differences between younger buyers, like millennials and Gen Z, and boomers?

"You would expect that because boomers have experienced many health plan enrollment seasons, the purchasing of a health plan would get easier over time," she says. "But that's not the case. Every time individuals change employers; they face a new signup process. If they lose their health benefits due to a job change or decide to become self-employed or they age into Medicare—the plan options available, the deductibles, the networks, the prices—all that changes. And plans are very different from one another, as are eligibility requirements and prices. An individual can go from being on a family plan through employer-sponsored coverage to each individual family member needing to be on a completely different plan. For example, a child with a permanent disability may need to go on Medicaid; a self-employed, single parent may need an individual plan; and a retired, but still working part-time, person may qualify for Medicare. None of these plans are the same in their designs, or in how you sign up for them.

"And while millennials are tech-savvy, they are industry-jargon challenged—perhaps even more so than the boomers! Millennials are also looking for plans with lower prices, wellness incentives, and app-based features and services. Gen Z may actually have a shot at an easier path to enrolling in a health plan.

They are more likely to align themselves with solutions—enrollment platforms—that do the heavy lifting and make enrolling in a health plan a simple and personalized click-through process: one phone, one thumb, and you're covered!"

RAY COSTANTINI, MD, CO-FOUNDER AND CEO OF BRIGHT.MD

If you read *The Digital Healthcare Revolution,* you may remember Dr. Ray Costantini and his company, Bright.md.

Ray is a pioneering healthcare executive, an innovative physician, and a seasoned entrepreneur who is passionate about making healthcare better. Prior to founding Bright.md, he led the design, build, deployment, and operations of three groundbreaking telehealth and digital health products at Providence Health and Services, one of the largest health systems in the country. He also previously founded three successful companies and is a national speaker on healthcare innovation, telehealth, and patient engagement.

In essence, Bright.md offers a new way for consumers to schedule appointments with their primary care providers, and to build ongoing relationships with them. In order to do so, Bright.md combines telehealth with a proprietary care automation platform. A secondary benefit, according to Bright.md, is that it "helps physicians and health systems provide more thorough and evidence-based remote diagnosis and treatment, along with a 15x improvement in efficiency."

Bright.md's unique selling proposition states, "The goal is to help health systems delight both their patients and providers, while improving clinical outcomes, dramatically lowering healthcare costs, and providing opportunities for new revenues. Bright.md is developing a new range of innovative technologies that include its #SmartExam, which the company describes as, 'your virtual physician.'"

Here is another part of their mission:

"The goal of Bright.md is to 'cut the cost of visits by 80 percent – while providing high-quality care patients love.'"

THE GROWTH OF BRIGHT.MD
BEFORE AND DURING COVID

During the pandemic years, Bright.md has grown exponentially. According to Ray, "We're more than twice the size that we were when we last talked, on multiple measures. We're now working with four of the 10 largest healthcare delivery systems in the country. We are pretty clearly the leading care automation platform that's out there.

"I think Covid really helped push healthcare to embrace telehealth. But more interesting things have happened too. Trends have forced healthcare as an industry to recognize the need for real digital transformation, and to consider the bigger question of how we can use technology to make healthcare better. How do we make it better for patients? How do we make it better for providers? How do we make it more affordable and accessible? How do we make it more connected?

"The result is changing where healthcare happens, which is nice. But it's resulting in largescale foundational challenges that healthcare is facing as a whole."

The pandemic turned just about everything upside-down in healthcare. Does the data that value-based care solutions like Bright.md generate help providers validate value-based care outcomes in a way that allows them to capture better remuneration? And how does that affect the providers' ability to deliver care in a meaningful way for the benefit of their patients?

Ray tells me, "In any value-based care setting, the target is to make the care that is delivered between 15 and 20 times more efficient. That's an easy conversation to have, and it is at our very core. This, in turn, makes care more affordable for patients. It makes it a more consistent experience for everybody involved. Our core value proposition is what delivers on that multiple aim of better outcomes, lower costs and a better experience for both patients and providers."

ON THE CHANGING ROLE OF TELEHEALTH

Bright.md doesn't even have a landline telephone for customers to connect with their company or schedule appointments with their caregivers.

Instead, Bright.md offers a platform that helps consumers find the kind of care they are looking for and need. To make that happen, Ray and his team are conceptualizing and building this capability every day, by focusing on key questions like:

- How can we gather all the right information?

- How can we empower the clinician?

- How can we remove all of the mundane administrative work that is clogging up the clinician's time so that we can put the humanity back into healthcare?

Ray summarizes, "How do we build the tools that make it so that the computer is working for the patients as the clinician, rather than the other way around?

"I don't know a single clinician who wouldn't say that 'Basically, I'm a slave to my EMR (Emergency Medical Records) system. It's not doing me any good. It has slowed my productivity down to the point where I am now spending 70 percent of my time on screens and keyboards, instead of with my patients.'"

Ray believes that situation is exacerbating provider burnout and inflating the costs of care and causing increased fragmentation across the whole spectrum of healthcare. But he also foresees that all the frustration in this area is providing incentives to make improvements. "We've got to be able to bring tools that are more comprehensive and that are really improving customers' access to care. We've got to be thinking about how we can deliver care differently and better."

RAY'S TAKE ON TELEHEALTH AS IT IS NOW

Ray believes that in the majority of instances, video interactions between physician and patient are not adding anything of clinical value to care.

"It doesn't help the clinician do anything differently," Ray says. "And that means that clinicians are doing the same amount of work. They're spending the same percentage of their time with patients as compared to with the computer. That's not where they want to be. It's not why they spent 25 years in school, to do data entry work. And those are the kinds of things that are causing provider burnout.

"And it doesn't help that they are still squeezing in 20 to 30 visits a day. It doesn't help that's all I have as a clinician to sell is 20-minute increments of my time. If you come in with a cold, I'm going to give you 20 minutes of my time. And if you come in with diabetes and congestive heart failure and COPD and a whole bunch of social determinant issues, you're still going to get about 20 minutes of my time.

"Realities like those are diminishing the quality of care, but they're not the primary issues. The primary issues come from this supply/demand issue and the fact that we have pushed clinicians to keep up with that demand and just do more. We just kept turning up the treadmill!

"By introducing tools that make the clinicians' job easier and better, we allow them to bring humanity and joy back into their work so that they're not on that treadmill all day long. They could actually be spending two minutes of their time for a simple condition. They have 40 minutes of time for complicated patients where they really want to be spending their time. Those are the kinds of things that can actually sustainably manage provider burnout which is now commonly recognized as one of healthcare's biggest threats. Everything else is a bandage."

WHAT HAPPENS NEXT?

"There have been a lot of corpses along the roadside to healthcare transformation," Ray says, "and companies like Google and Microsoft and Safeway and lots of folks have tried to transform the way that healthcare gets delivered.

"I am a lousy pundit, so I won't pretend to have the forward-looking answers, but I would say Amazon has taken on a lot of ambitious projects and they have had the infrastructure for what we need fora while. If I were a healthcare delivery system, I would be paying a lot of attention there. Walmart and all of those big box folks, they've got infrastructure. They've got consumer engagement. They've got financial motivations around foot traffic and prescriptions, and so on. The field is getting increasingly crowded, and your competition doesn't look like the bricks and mortar across the street from you anymore.

"And that to me...if it is healthcare delivery systems, they don't pay attention to that. If it's not this wave of transformation, there will be another and another. And another and another. It will happen. It is an inevitability. You can't avoid it. All you can do is delay using innovative new healthcare delivery models but that sounds an awful lot like Kodak and digital cameras. I don't think that's the game that anyone should be playing."

BEYOND TELEHEALTH LIES STILL MORE TECHNOLOGY

The really magical transformations will happen when we embrace the fact that advanced technologies across the board, not just telehealth, are changing the way healthcare is delivered and consumed. Those capabilities will make all aspects of healthcare, from primary care visits to management of payments and prescription medications, more efficient, more thorough, more accessible, more affordable, and using a word that Ray loves, more "delightful" for everybody involved.

I remember that at the HLTH19 conference, someone raised their hand and said, "I always thought of telehealth as a great way of managing social determinants of health. But it is not, it is furthering the divide." The message behind that comment was that we are making care more accessible for people who have coverage and who have everything at their fingertips already. But what about people who don't have access to that technology?

"I think video-based telehealth, as a specific example, is a model of concierge care," Ray says. "You are self-selecting as a group. You have access to Wi-Fi and a video camera. And you need all of those things. And it's not necessarily more affordable than in-person care. it is a model of convenience care. And there's nothing wrong with that. But we have to embrace what it is and what it's not. If you're on Medicaid and don't have a smartphone or computer or if you're in rural America and you have spotty 3G cell signal, video-based telehealth is not an option for you. We need to widen the digital divide, not narrow it."

MORE QUESTIONS EMERGE

My conversation with Ray begs the question, how do we keep moving forward? How do we continue making improvements every day, when roadblocks like the digital divide block the way? What can we expect next for this industry segment? And who is going to drive the change? Will it be innovators, or patients and consumers who will step up and say, "Can you see me? Can you meet me where I am? Can you give me what I need?"

Covid's dirty little secret is the depression-driven afflictions that come hand in hand with isolation. It isn't always easy to tell when someone is off just by looking at them. They may be a model of health from a weight perspective, even from an outward appearance of frame of mind. While Covid is not the only driver of depression and mental breakdowns, it is nice to have resources available to detect and manage those conditions.

SHEILA HAMILTON,
CEO OF BEYOND WELL SOLUTIONS

Sheila Hamilton is the CEO of Beyond Well Solutions. Her company provides a mental health solution for employers who want to engage employees in better behavioral health and wellness.

Sheila is a five-time Emmy-winning mental health journalist, and the author of *All the Things We Never Knew: Chasing the Chaos of Mental Illness*. Among the many awards she has won are the Ron Schmidt Community Service Award and the Judy Cushing Life Award for her advocacy for people with mental illness. She hosts the podcast *Beyond Well with Sheila Hamilton*.

As we have already noted, many healthcare innovators have chosen to work in the field because of a personal experience—an epiphany—that changed their lives. That was also the case with

Sheila. But her experiences were dramatically different from those of the other experts I interviewed for this book.

"I started the company because of my own experience in the mental health arena, which was with my husband, who was a very successful businessman," Sheila says. "At the age of 43, he started having very strange behaviors and was not motivated to run his company. He wasn't billing his clients and he was really starting to struggle.

"When I suggested that he go see a therapist, he was stigmatized by it. He'd grown up in a family that was just not willing to talk about mental health as something that was normal or something that we all struggle with. He was unwilling to accept the idea that we can all learn tools to deal with our anxiety. He was placed on the wrong medication and misdiagnosed because he didn't see a psychiatrist. He just went to a friend who was a physician and he spiraled downward. The day after he was let out of care, he died by suicide.

"I had been a reporter for almost 25 years and felt like I missed the biggest story of my life, which was how to identify people in mental health crises and what we can all do to help. It was then that I switched my journalism career for one that would allow me to develop content and programming that could help people realize we're all on a spectrum of mental health and we all need to have the tools and the resilience to be able to handle things that come up in our lives. We're all in need of mental health training. So that was the genesis for it."

Sheila is right. Mental health issues don't only affect people of specific demographics, they can affect anyone. Many of us encounter these problems and simply try to muscle through them. And Sheila points out that mental health challenges don't only affect people who are failing in their businesses and in their careers. These challenges can be experienced by highly successful people.

"It's important for people to understand that some of the

worst mental health crises in business affect people that are having their best life," she says. "These are people who are *there*. They have more customers than they've ever had before. They might be entrepreneurs who are really hitting big. But they're running out of the mental capacity to juggle everything that comes at them. They're not sleeping or eating well. They don't have someone that they can rely on to talk about their fears and their apprehension about the good stuff that's going on. And those people can go into a mental health crisis. We have to stop believing that mental health crises only afflict those who are genetically inclined toward depression.

"How do we cope with these problems? We soldier on. Some of us are more effective at it than others are. That is a big reason why we created our company to help solve this issue."

HOW MENTAL HEALTH
SUFFERED DURING THE PANDEMIC

Is it a fair call to say that mental health has been exacerbated by the Covid-19 pandemic? I asked Sheila and as you would expect, she was able to point me to relevant recent research.

She cited a recent Kaiser Permanente Family Foundation report that states that as the pandemic is drawing to a close, two-thirds of Americans reported high levels of anxiety and stress. In addition, seven in 10 employees state that the current work environment is "the most stressful time in their career." Those figures represent phenomenal increases from the last time that Kaiser reported on employees' mental health, prior to the pandemic. (For more information, view Kaiser's conclusions at business.kaiserpermanente.org.)

She also notes that younger workers have suffered a decline in mental health. Roughly four out of 10 workers report not being able to cope on a daily basis with the demands of remote work and cited increased levels of anxiety and depression.

"It was a crisis," Sheila states. "And I think if you didn't have your own existential crisis about what it meant to have a worldwide pandemic, you probably weren't paying attention."

To address those problems among the working population, Beyond Well created employer programs that connected employees with psychiatrists, psychologists, social workers, and others. And the programs created included additional services for employees who were dealing with the specific challenges of schooling children at home, and also with employees who were experiencing trauma during the time of the protests following the murder of George Floyd.

Interestingly enough, Sheila notes that alongside their employees, success-oriented C-suite-level executives were among the people who were really hit hard. Many of them were asking deeper questions like, "What am I doing with my life?" and "What is my real purpose?"

But Sheila notes that positive change has resulted from the pandemic too. Companies have become more open to discussing and addressing the anxieties and worries that employees face every day.

Sheila says, "That elephant has been in the room for a long, long time. The pandemic brought things to the point where we cannot ignore him."

CREATING A REVOLUTION
IN COMPANY WELLNESS AND WELLBEING

How does Beyond Well Solutions work with companies to offer employees—from the top down—access to the wellness programs Sheila and her team have developed?

They have worked with the HR departments at large and

small companies to make sure that employees know what kind of help is available. But Sheila believes that merely being available is not enough.

For mental health to become part of what a company does—and what its culture is—Sheila has noted that orientation toward mental wellness needs to be a top-down initiative. In some companies, employees through the ranks don't fully trust that company leaders and top executives genuinely believe in mental-health initiatives. And when that trust is lacking, employees may hesitate to take part in the programs. They can also be afraid that their privacy is being violated if they take part. Some employees are even afraid that they will lose their jobs if they admit to depression or anxiety.

What is the solution? One is for company leaders to talk about their own worries and anxieties, not to conceal them. And something else, according to Sheila: "There has to be an organic and very, very vulnerable and open conversation with radical empathy for what people are going through while they try to navigate this period."

HOW EMPLOYEES ENCOUNTER AND EXPERIENCE BEYOND WELLNESS PROGRAMS

Let's say you are an employee who needs counseling—perhaps you are experiencing anxiety or stress. How will you learn about the Beyond Wellness programs your company makes available, and what will the services you access be like?

As Sheila noted above, people are more willing to seek out and take part if company leaders are open and accepting of the fact that employees might need assistance. She also notes that company communications can play a critical role.

Companies can distribute weekly updates and resource materials on pertinent topics like the challenges of raising school-age children during the post-pandemic period. Some of the content can be in the form of videos that address particular concerns that employees could be dealing with.

"Employees can discover a video or lesson on a topic that addresses their needs, click on it, and watch what they need," Sheila says. "Plus, the resources can be siloed so that if an employee has a child who is experiencing anxiety, that employee can jump there and find advice.

"What we like about this approach is that it doesn't require people to sit in front of a screen and watch content that doesn't pertain to what they need. People are really fatigued with sitting in front of videos and being tethered to a laptop can cause even more stress."

But with the right formatting and presentation of helpful material, Sheila believes people can become more of what she calls, "the CEOs of their own mental health."

The result can be employees who are happier, more productive, and better able to deal with the challenges of what it is like to work today. This approach will save companies money too.

"We never want employees to get to the point where they check into the ER to deal with an issue that pertains to mental health," Sheila says. "We want companies to become involved much earlier so that never happens—and so that employees are happier and better adjusted to working for companies that care about their wellbeing."

Beyond Wellness is undertaking initiatives that can cultivate healthier employees, happier companies and overall, a happier workforce in our country as the pandemic fades into memory.

INSIGHTS AND PREDICTIONS
FROM ANN MOND JOHNSON, CEO,
AMERICAN TELEMEDICINE ASSOCIATION

Ann Mond Johnson joined the American Telemedicine Association (ATA) as CEO in 2018. Her experience includes building, launching and leading client-driven companies that have been innovators in healthcare technology and data to support consumers using healthcare.

Prior to joining the ATA, Ann served as CEO of Zest Health, a technology-enabled service; as board chair and advisor to ConnectedHealth, a leading provider of private insurance exchanges; and as co-founder and CEO of Subimo, a pioneer in healthcare cost and quality decision support tools for consumers. Ann began her career in healthcare data and information as senior vice president at Sachs Group (now part of IBM Watson/ Truven Health). She also worked at a multi-hospital system in Minneapolis which is now part of Allina.

Ann's ability to inspire and lead diverse teams has helped build both profitable organizations and innovation in the industry. Widely acknowledged as a thought leader, she presents at a range of professional meetings and conferences. She also maintains an active professional network and affiliations, including membership in the Healthcare Executive Leadership Network and Women Business Leaders of the U.S. Healthcare Industry Foundation. Ann served on the Healthcare Advisory Council for UMB Bank and as an advisor to several start-ups. She was inducted into the Chicago Entrepreneurship Hall of Fame in 2016.

Ann's involvement also extends to non-profit service organizations, including serving on the board of Round Earth Media, a non-profit organization focused on journalism (now part of the International Women's Media Foundation). She is a member of the

Ambassadors Council for N Street Village in Washington, D.C., and currently serves on the board of Pathfinder International, a non-profit organization committed to countrywide solutions to achieve universal sexual and reproductive health and rights.

ON THE GROWING USE OF TELEHEALTH

"I think that the thing that came out of this pandemic is a confirmation that once people used telehealth or virtual services, they would like them," Ann says. "It was just a question of getting them to use it. And that's exactly what happened.

"It's like, oh my God, this actually works! And so consumers were pleasantly surprised. The other thing that came out of it was that they said they would use it again. From the convenience and lower costs in many instances, to just the whole avoidance of time wasted. That proved to be an important thing from the consumer's vantage point. And likewise, from the provider's vantage point."

ANN IS RIGHT!

Not only is telehealth easy, but it offers immediate benefits that people will continue to rely upon in the years ahead. Consumers are saying, "I didn't have to get up and leave my home to go to appointments, because my smartphone is able to connect me. This has a meaningful benefit for me, and moreover, it solved a real-world healthcare problem."

But Ann points out that people didn't immediately adopt, accept and love telehealth. Some consumers were actually "terrified" of using it. One cause of that fear, she feels, is that people believed that they had been cut loose from their resources of expert guidance and direction. They were using their apps, for example, and going here and there to access advice and care, but who was saying that the sources they found were the best or correct ones?

What overcame that fear and those objections?

"I think that it was not just the video visits that worked, but the element of asynchronous interactions where consumers would ask questions and get answers they were looking for. They would find, for example, that what they were experiencing was not symptomatic with Covid."

But they also got another layer of advice. One example? They would be given advice like, "Here's where you are, but if things change here are the next steps you should follow." People found that new telehealth platforms gave them guidance and immediate feedback.

Ann takes this line of thinking further.

"Digital health saved the day," she says, "It saved the healthcare system from imploding."

CASE STUDY: ADOPTION TRENDS FOR TELEHEALTH

"One of my favorite stories about telehealth is about a pediatrician here in D.C.," says Ann. "And because she was older, she was assigned to, and belonged to, a group of pediatricians. They were doing well, conducting child checkups digitally and virtually. She was thrilled.

"She was able to accomplish a lot. She couldn't do the immunizations or the vaccines, but she could do a lot of other things. And that was pleasant and surprising for her. It was incredibly reassuring for parents too.

"What we are doing now is collecting these stories as part of a campaign to ensure that the gains that we've made stick at both a federal and state level."

ON LAWS AND REGULATIONS
AFFECTING TELEHEALTH USAGE

One underlying issue that Ann has noticed is that regulations have not caught up with what technology can do. And if you look at a lot of the regulations that were in place that have now been waived or relaxed during the pandemic, we see that some of them were sort of absurd. As Ann defines it, there has been so much architecture and scaffolding.

The problem with these structures is that they are about providing ease and increased profits not for the patient, but for other entities within the universe of healthcare—insurers, plan administrators, and others.

They are not there to protect the patient. The fact that you have to drive somewhere in order to get care wasn't helping anyone. And so that was something that had been a target for a long time to eliminate.

"To our delight and surprise," Ann says, "our representatives in government do want to ensure that Americans get care where and when they need it, and they want to ensure that it's safe and it's effective and it's appropriate, and we do want to enable clinicians to do more good for more people. I will tell you that the new administration is very engaged, very involved, very supportive of telehealth. And we were gratified by that. There's a very strong bipartisan coalition on the Hill. I have an interview next week with Congressmen Glenn Thompson and David Schweikert. They're all in with telehealth and that's exciting."

ENABLERS AND SUPPORTERS

Ann points out that corporations like HP, Sony and Microsoft all have commitments to telehealth development.

"And she adds, "I think that what we're seeing now—because we've put together comments from the physician—we've seen some really important developments or heroes that came out of this pandemic that we hope to get incorporated going forward.""

YET WE ARE STILL CATCHING UP

"We're going to make mistakes," Ann says, "so it could be a situation where a physician gets off the phone with a patient and says, 'Oh, no, you have to come in.'

"In that instance, which is the starkest characterization of what can happen that is inefficient, patients are going to doubt how well telehealth is working. There is always going to be a transition period that we're going to have to go through."

Ann is right, there are always going to be obstacles we have yet to overcome. We have to continue moving forward, recognizing that there are different layers of protection and safeguarding that we want to see maintained and strengthened.

"There are certainly things that we have to work through," Ann says. But telehealth? "This trend is already in place and the train has left the station."

ABNER MASON,
FOUNDER AND CEO, CONSEJOSANO

You may remember Abner Mason from *The Digital Health Revolution*. He has additional insights about using telehealth and other tools to make excellent healthcare available to the underserved people in our country. ConsejoSano remains nothing short of inspiring.

Abner Mason is the founder and CEO of ConsejoSano, the only patient engagement and care navigation solution designed to help clients activate their multicultural patient and member populations to better engage with the healthcare system. ConsejoSano's clients are typically health plans and provider groups serving Medicaid and Medicare Advantage members and patient populations.

ConsejoSano utilizes multilingual, multi-channel engagement (two-way SMS, voice, etc.) along with culturally relevant messaging to increase engagement. ConsejoSano helps clients lower costs and improve health outcomes related to care for multicultural populations that face cultural, language, and social challenges in accessing care. Through healthcare navigators that provide in-language support, ConsejoSano builds trust with at-risk patients and steers them to more effective self-care and utilization of their healthcare benefits.

Abner is also founder and co-chair of HealthTech 4 Medicaid (www.HT4M.org), a non-profit organization for CEOs building innovative solutions for the Medicaid market. Abner previously served as founder and CEO of the Workplace Wellness Council of Mexico (www.wwpcmex.com). With 152 current clients including 40 multi-nationals, the Mexico council is now the leading workplace wellness company in Mexico. From 2002 - 2009, Abner served as founder and executive director of AIDS Responsibility Project, where he created the first business councils on HIV/AIDS in Mexico and Jamaica. Abner was also appointed by President George W. Bush to the Presidential Advisory Council on HIV/AIDS. He served as chairman of the International Committee from 2002 - 2005. Abner also served as chief policy advisor, chief secretary, and undersecretary of transportation and construction for Massachusetts Governors Paul Cellucci and Jane Swift from 1997 - 2002. Abner has dedicated his life and work to making superior healthcare available to everyone.

ABNER TALKS ABOUT CONSEJOSANO

"Our name means 'healthy advice' in Spanish. We are a patient engagement and patient navigation company with a social mission. We believe that everybody deserves high-quality healthcare, regardless of what they look like, where they come from or frankly, what their income is.

"I became founder and CEO because I saw a problem that we have with our health system in the U.S. And that problem was getting worse, not better. And the problem is that our country has changed over the last four to five decades and become dramatically more multicultural. But our healthcare system hasn't kept up with that demographic change, and that demographic change is pretty extraordinary.

"For example, California is today a majority-minority state. So is Texas. The whole country will become majority-minority, according to the last census. We'll hit that in 2050."

CHANGING AMERICA

Abner believes we are on a path as a nation. There is no changing it. But we do have a choice. Our healthcare system was designed to serve primarily English speakers and primarily people who could pay for care.

Our established system works quite well if you are a traditional English speaker and you're in a higher income bracket. But our country has changed and because our healthcare system hasn't kept up, we have a mismatch between the healthcare system and the people it is supposed to serve. And ConsejoSano is determined to fix that. We shouldn't just stand by and watch it and see this problem getting worse and worse. We need to take action to address it.

And that's what ConsejoSano is doing. Abner and his organization are trying to use technology and data to help its plan partners or clients, bridge that gap.

ON THE BIG PICTURE

"You've got healthcare," Abner tells me. "You got healthcare stakeholders, like health systems and health plans, who are good people. They want to serve all of their members. They just don't know how. And their members have become so diverse in terms of being multicultural, meaning coming from different cultures and speaking different languages and having a totally different understanding of healthcare and how they engage with healthcare. Health plans and other healthcare stakeholders are struggling to figure out how to engage with those multicultural members.

"Then on top of that layer, we have also found out in the last decade in particular, that the factors that drive healthcare are not all determined in the clinician's office. In fact, just the opposite, much of what drives and determines a person's healthcare are the factors that that person experiences outside of the clinical setting.

"We call these the social determinants of health. But we have a better understanding now that there are many other factors—nonclinical factors—that need to be taken into account. And our healthcare system, the way it was set up, is not well equipped to serve multicultural people, it's not well equipped to address social determinants of health."

Abner's assessment is correct. If you step back and look at it, we have some real challenges with our healthcare system. It needs to change, and the status quo is not sufficient. And what he calls "little bitty steps" aren't enough. We need to think boldly about how we make our healthcare system work for the country that we've become and how we can address the problems that the people of the country actually have.

This mission is incredibly ambitious. But let's view it through the lens of what has happened during the time of Covid-19.

THE IMPACT OF THE PANDEMIC

"Due to the pandemic," Abner says, "ConsejoSano was able to generate 50,000 telehealth visits, in a matter of only three months. We found that, interestingly, doctors prefer video visits because they can use them to get a lot of information about patients' health concerns and issues. But we also learned that patients today prefer a call.

"The pandemic forced the stakeholders to tear down their walls and silos and to actually think about what was good for the patient, which is good, and to align the payment with what was right for the patient. The situation changed quickly. Many providers didn't discriminate between telehealth and telemedicine, they simply needed to deliver care.

"That's a very important thing that we need to have going forward, in terms of policy. I believe that we should treat patients more like consumers and let them have a voice in how they communicate. If they prefer a call, we ought to let them have a call. And we ought not discriminate in terms of reimbursement. The system is going to try to shift people over to where providers get paid more."

THE WORLD TURNED "UPSIDE DOWN"

"The pandemic turned our world upside down," Abner says. "Overall, it's been a terrible tragedy. About 600,000 Americans are dead. Americans have reported nearly 33 million infections. If you look around the world, the numbers are just horrifying. And that doesn't account for people who are infected but got well. An undetermined number of those people will suffer in the future, because as we're finding out now, some people have residual impacts from the virus.

"Our economy was turned upside down. Education has been fundamentally changed. There is no question it has overall been a nightmare that we have all been living through. But I think there have been some silver linings, because for so many years, healthcare in America has been ossified. It is hard to change healthcare. Even when technology comes along, our healthcare system is resistant to using those changes. One of the silver linings of the Covid crisis in healthcare is that the whole system had to be open to disruption in a way that it hadn't been before. There was no choice. I am talking specifically here about telehealth. We've struggled in this country mightily to get that technology broadly used. It's better. It's cheaper. It's easier for the patients. It helps close gaps in care. Often, in terms of disparities in rural versus urban regions.

"There are a lot of enormous benefits to telehealth. But we couldn't get all of the stakeholders aligned before the pandemic because people had their own interests and protected their turf and their incomes. There are many fiefdoms in healthcare. And the pandemic forced everyone to kind of say, 'OK, at least for now, we've got to act like healthcare is more important as opposed to protecting our interests and our fiefdoms.'

"But people didn't stop being human beings because the pandemic started. They had all the health issues they had always had. They still needed healthcare.

"Let's incentivize the entire system. Let's treat patients like consumers, let them pick the way they want to communicate and then don't have a differential payment scheme. One of the more subtle benefits was that it included lower-income people. We proved without a doubt that they will use these new technologies if given the chance."

USING TECHNOLOGY TO BUILD TRUST

Abner points out that trust is the force that makes most everything else work in the world of healthcare. He believes that the most critical question about technology is, how do you use it to build trust with patients and end users?

"Only when you have built trust can you expect that that patient will listen to you and take action based on what you've said to them," he says. "So, figure out a way to communicate that builds that trust so that you can then have a real open and honest conversation. The result of that conversation is that patient taking an action and participating in their recovery in an informed way.

"That's what we're doing at ConsejoSano. We spend all of our time trying to do this. And we're trying to do it with some of the hardest-to-reach patients or membership plan member populations because they are multicultural, they're low income, they have very high levels of distrust or lack of trust. We have found that as we have looked at all the different ways to try to engage the patient, is that the most effective is to try to build a relationship based on what we call culture. Specifically, that patient's culture. We collect a lot of data, public and private data as well as claims data.

"We add to that deep understanding of how different communities in our country engage healthcare. What are the social determinants in their life that either make it easier or harder for them to get healthcare? What are their fears? What is in the back of their heads when they hear the word 'doctor'? If you use real world healthcare data and then detail what that allows us to do for a given population that we want to engage, that is how we build what we call a cultural cohort.

"That explains why we have built a technology platform that allows us to micro-segment the larger population into much smaller groups, based on culture. We then design our engagement strategy, including content based on that cultural cohort. We are not treating everybody the same.

"Then there is the question of translation. Sometimes a company where people speak English just translate their messaging into 13 different languages and send it out. That approach does not work. But that is what healthcare in America today does. That kind of language-based translation only tells people that they aren't important. Often times, we don't even get the grammar and diction right, so we lose credibility coming right out of the gates.

"We don't have to treat people that way anymore. What it says is that who you are as a patient doesn't really matter, because I'm sending you the same message as I'm sending someone whose life experience is completely different. The only thing I've done is translate it, usually not well. The most important things that make them who they are aren't important. You should not be surprised if they say, 'I'm not too interested in talking to you because you have told me who I am doesn't matter.'"

Ever wonder how to keep people engaged? If healthcare still has an Achilles' heel, this is it. GoMo Health is poised to become the next most important company you have never heard of.

BOB GOLD EXPLAINS
FUNDAMENTAL CONSUMER MOTIVATIONS

Bob Gold is CEO of GoMo Health, an innovative New Jersey-based company that is a leader in designing, implementing, and marketing award-winning, personalized patient engagement solutions that support the continuum of care.

Bob and his team have developed what they call Behavioral Rx, which they describe as a scalable and cost-effective way that companies can use to engage with end-users that enables better self-management, healthy decisions, and improved outcomes.

GoMo is a bit like the Wizard of Oz—an engaged entity that is always out of sight yet is working its engagement magic for other companies. You can't download a GoMo app and use it on your phone. If you are an end-user or a consumer of healthcare services, you might be interacting with a company that employs GoMo solutions and never even see its name.

What GoMo does, in essence, is to help consumer engagement experiences for customers who use the services of other healthcare companies. Bob Gold is a positively brilliant man who has spent his life studying and codifying what makes consumers want to engage with companies. His clients span healthcare's value chain of health plans, providers and innovators.

As I spoke with him, I was thinking about Maslow's famous hierarchy of needs—the underlying needs, identified by a Russian psychologist named Abraham Maslow—that are supposed to be the main human needs that motivate people to act. Bob, in his way, has identified a parallel set of human motivations.

We'll take a look at those in a few paragraphs. But first, let's get an overview of the current healthcare landscape that Bob and all the other companies outlined in this book are constrained to work within.

THE HIGH VIEW

We are now a decade into the age of the Affordable Care Act. Coincidentally, we are also 10 years into the digital healthcare revolution.

Since then we have seen about $50 billion invested in technologies that were essentially intended to help us manage chronic conditions across all populations of health.

But despite that level of investment, there are still gaps that are not being adequately addressed. Mental health and addiction assistance are two of them.

Why are those gaps still there?

Bob has an opinion: "It's because we suck at engaging and interacting with people. I don't care if you're a provider or a health plan, you simply don't know how to reach out and touch somebody in a way that doesn't irritate them. You don't elicit the level of participation from them that they need."

WHY END-USERS DON'T FULLY ENGAGE IN HEALTHCARE

"The way healthcare has traditionally delivered its products," Bob tells me, "it does not provide any cognitive or behavioral value.

"In many cases, it only adds to anxiety, stress, and cognitive overload. Therefore, whether healthcare is delivered either in person or via technology, it reduces feelings of self-efficacy. That's the short answer I can give about what is wrong with the way that healthcare providers engage with consumers."

LESSONS FROM LEARNING TO PLAY THE PIANO

Why do healthcare providers fail to engage end-users to participate actively and effectively in their own care?

"Let's say that a consumer has just been diagnosed with type 2 diabetes," Bob says. "Let's further say that you're that consumer. You were just in the hospital, where you got diagnosed, and then you got released. Or maybe you just got diagnosed with asthma or heart disease.

"You go home, you're frightened. You need guidance. But what happens next? You get told to come back to see the physician who diagnosed you, maybe in a month, or two months, or three. And when you go back, your appointment is squeezed into a little time slot. And you leave just as confused, and probably just as frightened, as you were when you first were diagnosed. You still aren't sure what to do, much less when and why.

"Let's compare that to the way a person learns how to play the piano. You first get an expert teacher who sits with you. And they actually play and then they sit with you, and you play, and they correct you in that moment and you do it again in that moment, and then they watch you and then they meet with you again, and they watch you again and help you take corrective measures. It is intimate and it is interactive.

"Now, let's return to that situation in which you just found out you're a type 2 diabetic. The doctor gave you instructions and now you're on your own. No one is watching what you do. It makes no sense. Unless you are connecting the mind and the body, providing guidance and understanding on an intimate basis, it is impossible to get patients to change their outlook or build their confidence and trust themselves and find themselves capable. They need help when they need it not when we want to provide it to them.

"If that physician is a top endocrinologist, he or she knows the things that a patient should do. But that physician is not there to explain what those behaviors are or to say to the patient, 'I have seen you do what you need to do, and you have the knowledge and skills you need to succeed.'"

THE WEDDING PLANNER ANALOGY

Bob offers another analogy, comparing planning a wedding to managing a health condition or disease.

"Imagine you're planning a wedding and you go to a wedding planner who says, 'Oh, no, I only do the first part of the wedding, what happens in the chapel. If you want a reception, you need another planner for that. You want flowers? You need a third wedding planner for that. And music? I don't do that either.'

"Yet this is precisely the structure we are told is acceptable in healthcare. You see a primary care doctor and then, maybe you are told you then need to see a cardiologist or a psychiatrist or an oncologist. You know how it works. And while it makes sense to have special teams, what you need is a digital, therapeutic or engagement program that integrates those experiences into a singular care experience for an individual, like what a real-world wedding planner does. He or she manages all these different experiences and makes it a single experience for you. And that is where we need to be going in the world of healthcare."

ATM machines offer additional insights.

"People go to an ATM machine, and they stick in their little card," Bob says. "And they enter their PIN, and they transact their business. They don't have to get to know the bank, or understand where the cash is stored, or how it appears. Yet again, in the world of healthcare, people have been taught that they need to understand and manage all those separate processes."

CAPTURING IMPORTANT DATA

Providers don't own patients' data. So how do they get those patients to provide it?

Bob says, "It's actually extremely simple to do when you apply behavioral science to it. There are things you need to do to get someone to be reciprocal. The first is shared decision-making. The second is that you have to adjust to, and reflect, the lifestyle of the patient."

BUILDING COMPLIANCE TO CARE ROUTINES

Bob opines that providers often have little understanding of why people listen to them or whether they will strictly follow their care recommendations. Why is that?

"Basically, you have to earn the right," Bob says. "If you can get that individual to accept you as a credible source, which means that they believe you understand them, then all of a sudden they will take your recommendations to heart.

"But why do people continue adhering and taking part in their own recovery? It is because you are providing great content and great information that addresses their personal situation and needs. When people decide not to follow your recommendations anymore, when they think what you are offering is not for them, that's usually because you've didn't ask the right questions.

"They get into a position where they haven't taken a medication in three months. But you keep sending reminders. You don't understand them at all because you have never asked about them. They think that you, as a provider, have no idea who they are."

CHAPTER NINE
WHERE DOES CONNECTED HEALTH TAKE US NEXT?

Looking back on the last ten years, you get a profound sense of excitement for what the stodgy, buttoned-down healthcare industry has accomplished. You also get a sense of angst that in spite of all our improvements to healthcare, there is still much to be done.

If you haven't figured it out by now, I am a huge fan of building on our incremental wins. While many argue about whether the glass is half full or half empty, I will argue tooth and nail that the glass has always been full…half water, half air! Still, every now and then, it is breathtaking to simply appreciate what a ride it has been. We have seen over $50 billion invested in exciting new healthcare technologies since the dawn of the Affordable Care Act. With that, there have been some absolutely amazing benefits and some equally spectacular failures. When companies like Virta Health are touting they have now reversed type 2 diabetes for more than 50,000 customers, how can you help but marvel at that and ask, what's next? While we are shopping for benefits and noticing the industry services our needs, we sense that we have taken a giant step toward becoming a more consumer-like experience. In spite of that, one of our most humbling failures has come from a very new participant with consumer DNA that was expected to disrupt and change the industry but didn't—Haven, probably the most hyped new healthcare entrant that quickly became a nonentity. Experiences like that drive home the point that healthcare is complex, opaque, and difficult to navigate.

Don't feel bad if you don't remember Haven; they were the company that never was. When Amazon, Berkshire Hathaway and JP Morgan all came together, they were hailed as a super company that would change the industry and there was much fanfare.

Yet, like Safeway Health before them, they discovered a simple and harsh truth—controlling costs is a lot easier when you are doing it internally and can control all your variables. It becomes a slippery slope when you try to bottle that and monetize it.

We have heard profound insights from all of our thought leaders in this book, but one sentiment echoed by Brad Fluegel and Torben Nielsen stands out—we don't live in the healthcare world, we live in the real world. We have jobs, children to care for, long commutes and shopping to do. In a world where two-income households have become the norm, we simply don't have time to become healthcare experts, nor do we see value in learning the jargon. While patients, health plan members and consumers have all proven that they will engage, they still lack knowledge on what to connect with and why.

Our consumption model is still dominated by an employer-provided benefits model, meaning we probably only know about what our employers have pre-selected for us. This model has created a fundamental dynamic that has long worked against making any real improvements to our system; health plans don't have a consumer heritage and they aren't always good about communicating their innovations, much less how you can benefit from using them.

Healthcare is a participative sport. Consumers not only have to advocate for ourselves when it comes to getting the very best care possible, we have to "own" the state of our own health and do everything we can to maintain good health. Fortunately, we are learning how to get and stay connected. How do you have a voice when your only interaction with your health plan is when they mess up your claim? Further to that, when the only time you interact with your provider is when there is something wrong? Writing It Takes a Village reminded me about what prompted me to start writing about healthcare in the first place. What good is all this innovation if nobody knows about it?

I often tell people about a conversation I had with a couple of old schoolmates who confided in me that they both now have type 2 diabetes. When I asked them if they had ever heard of Virta or Omada Health, much less Noom—tools that can put them in touch with clinicians, nutritionists, and caregivers—they both said "No, nobody cares about us, we did this to ourselves." If the secret to better caring for people is meeting them where they are, then we are still failing miserably. Digital health capabilities are useless if people don't know about them.

Probably two of the more subtle and nuanced benefits of what I have come to call "The Digital Health Revolution" are these. First, health plans for the first time ever have been forced to work directly with consumers. Second, because of the marketplaces and exchanges, health plans are finally developing a consumer approach, treating you like you are their customer and not an employee. Not only does this apply to how you shop and select your plan, but how you schedule and pay for your healthcare services. Whenever I hear people pontificate on the politics of healthcare, regardless of whether they are pro or con ACA, I often wonder if they ever think about this. Health plans are treating us like customers and not simply a nuisance for whom they process claims.

The other interesting dynamic, and this one is only now emerging, is that for the first time in the history of healthcare, we seem ready to address the real root causes of bad health. The very term healthcare is a bit of a misnomer. It has always meant sick care, and there was very little incentive to change that. Let's face it, the more times you visit your doctor, the more that doctor made. Yet we have been transitioning toward a model that rewards care givers for delivering real value. Rewarding for better health outcomes has been a godsend.

This notion of addressing root causes is exemplified in the writings of California's Surgeon General Dr. Nadine Burke Harris who pioneered the concept of Adverse Childhood Experiences (ACE) scoring. Dr. Harris bravely opened a clinic in one of San Francisco's impoverished neighborhoods only to have that epiphany moment when she realized that improving access to care doesn't move the needle as much as you might think. Understanding the drivers of poor health, be they social determinants or hereditary, are keys. I came up with a tagline at my first digital health company: "You can't manage what you don't measure." You also can't truly eradicate healthcare issues without better understanding what is creating them.

Those two simple things alone are enough to get excited about the direction we are going in healthcare.

Whenever I keynote at healthcare conferences and industry events, I always message where we are now this way:

- Digital Health 1.0 was when we disproved the popular myth that people won't engage.

- Digital Health 2.0 was when big data and "quantified self" gave rise to predictive analytics. There seemed to be a device or app for everything.

- Digital Health 3.0 is when "connected health" becomes the new norm, and our health data becomes actionable in near real-time.

This model of engaging, analyzing and then acting on our health data is forcing a new mindset around what needs to better connect to healthcare. Fortunately, the technology architecture that has evolved is ideally suited for better connecting us in a meaningful way while delivering measurable value. Digital health didn't start out that way. The EMR (Electronic Medical Records) segment began life as proprietary databases where sharing wasn't a core element of the design. If a patient wanted a second opinion or even to see a specialist helping them with a procedure, that provider needed to be using the same EMR as the referring doctor or that patient was tough out of luck.

So, what is it that needs to better connect to healthcare and how does this help us manage the issue of root causes? As Austin Beutner or the Angeles Unified School District shared with us, what we teach our children in our schools about nutrition and exercise matters. Workout facilities with state-of-the-art machinery and electronics for tracking our progress are every bit as important as gym classes and after-school sports. We can't feed our children sugar-based lunches and provide them with candy-filled vending machines and then pretend that this doesn't contribute to the obesity problems our children will have later in life. As it turns out, schools can be an excellent line of defense when it comes to helping us manage issues associated with social determinants of health. We have finally reached a point where we are realizing that social services and mental health resources are just as important as college counseling.

As we go to print, the new shiny-object, white-hot segment of healthcare is what is being called F.A.M. or "Food as Medicine." Healthcare has suddenly discovered that good nutrition is a fundamental pillar of good health. What took us so long? Some would argue that without CMS regulation making meals reimbursable, F.A.M. would never take off, but today healthy meals are covered by your Medicare Advantage plan.

COVID has been a big driver in making meal delivery mainstream. While many are focusing on specialty diets that help us manage chronic conditions like diabetes and hypertension, how long will it be before meal delivery is something that everyone is offered under their healthcare plan? EatFitGo, GA Foods, Mom's Meals and Freshly are all flexing their muscles and they all have clout. Eating healthy is becoming subscription-based. As you surround that with digital health tools from Noom, who is leveraging behavioral and cognitive principles to drive the psychological approach, you connect what you eat to how you feel in a track-able way that allows for timely interventions and education along the way. It's 100 percent digital, and with you at all times. It helps you track what you eat and when you eat it to better manage your weight and power you through dark periods. Before I started using Noom, I didn't realize I would frequently snack because I was just plain bored. My tendency to eat when bored led to additional pounds. Additional pounds led to knee and back problems. Knee and back problems led to working out less and losing energy, and losing energy invited the potential for depression. If you are getting a sense that this is all circular and connected, then go to the head of the class. Elo recognizes that there is nothing more personal than your diet and has built an entire company around providing important supplements that are tailored to you, based on your biometrics, to help you optimize your calorie burn. Finally, you have companies like Jenny Craig with a business model that now includes coaching, meal delivery and more. Probably the nicest thing about these new emerging tools is that they were designed from the ground up to become your tools. What a refreshing change from tools designed specifically for getting your doctor paid faster or letting your health plan determine what is best for you. Finally, the industry is putting your needs first.

Probably no healthcare industry segment has been more fun to track than retail. Roughly 75 percent of the U.S. population lives within five miles of a Walgreens or CVS. Each of these retailers have chosen a different path to earn our business. CVS Health is integrating pharmacy and health plans to better optimize your experience and provide cost savings. Their goal is to own their value chain and better control costs. Walgreens has taken a decidedly different approach, pursuing joint ventures and best-of-breed partnerships that deliver a total wellness approach to health. When you walk past a Walgreens, you might get "nudged" by Vim to step inside to see a Jenny Craig nutritionist to help you manage your hypertension. A doctor at VillageMD might even prescribe a meal plan for you that your health insurer will cover. Krogers can either start preparing your healthy meal choices for you to pick up at the store or deliver healthy ingredients right to your door. If you are too busy to shop, Jenny Craig will deliver you a meal to your home and your health plan will cover it,-because your meal was prescribed by a doctor. Walgreens is determined to get out in front of our sick-care trappings by focusing on a comprehensive set of solutions designed to help you get and stay healthy. What an evolution from simply going in to pick up your prescription and maybe buying supplements or devices.

In the Pacific Northwest, an exciting new brand of retail health is emerging at ZoomCare. I am never sure whether to describe them as tech-savvy providers or provider-savvy technologists. They have a propensity for developing their own solutions because they believe they are in a position to better understand precisely what their patients and customers need than any third-party vendor. They are bringing this clinical experience to employers, making it easy to get access to quality healthcare right at work. They also have a heart. Their "free care" night in impoverished neighborhoods throughout the Pacific Northwest is as inspirational a story as you will find in healthcare.

Yet, in spite of all this, we still have entire populations of health falling through the cracks and this is where organizations like ConsejoSano fit in. They are by no means the only organization dedicated to making sure those who need care get it. More often than not, it is an immigrant community where English is the second language, so navigating the complexities of healthcare in their new home is even more challenging. Monument Impact in the San Francisco Bay Area does the same.

If retail health is redefining healthcare and taking the concept of meeting you where you are to new levels, then homecare isn't far behind. Look for the next trend in healthcare to focus on delivering hospital-level care right in your home. Homecare is evolving from elderly care and end-of-life hospice to better manage post discharge challenges and help us with mental health and physical therapy. Even oncology care is now being delivered at home. Devices are reducing the friction of keeping us connected. If you have Wi-Fi, then connecting is easy. Your sleep and activity can now be tracked by wearing an Oura ring on your finger. Nutrition can be calibrated in real time by exhaling into a Lumen. Apple makes all this data harvestable so each app can store and later use the data you have chosen to share with it, providing a more comprehensive view of who you are, how you feel and what you do. My first digital health company would express that with a simple health score. Leveraging gaming principals had us aiming for a higher score.

Not everything is an app or a platform. Some of these technologies don't even require a registration process or web portal to log onto. In fact, the trend of the future is that we won't even know we are using a digital health tool at all. Walgreens for example is using Vim to nudge you toward a nutritionist to help you with your diet challenges.

We can access healthcare while we are out shopping, checking apps on our phone, and now, while we are at home. The more we push healthcare to meet us where we are, the more we appreciate that can mean meeting us anywhere.

And another trend is evolving quickly:

We want to recuperate and heal at home, not in hospitals or other care facilities.

People want to get out of the hospital earlier to be with their loved ones and be near the things they hold most dear. There are many reasons why getting released from hospitals earlier simply makes sense:

- *From the consumer's perspective . . .* People want to get back home to normal routines and recuperating at home costs much less than recuperating in a hospital.

- *From the hospital's perspective . . .* It makes operational and financial sense to allow patients to go home as early as possible while helping to manage the discharge risk.

- *From the insurer's perspective . . .* It saves money to have patients arrive home as quickly as possible and recuperate there. It also keeps members connected to their care providers.

Getting care at home is not only about what happens after leaving the hospital. It also applies to people who simply want to age in place or deal with chronic conditions while living at home.

YET THERE ARE ISSUES TO ADDRESS

Patients want to be sure that going home, or staying home, is a safe thing to do. Hospitals do not want to expose themselves to legal risks that can result from releasing patients early. And insurers, from their side of the situation, realize that releasing patients too soon can result in hospital readmissions, health complications, and opening up a Pandora's box of problems that they hoped to avoid by releasing patients early in the first place. So, what to do?

The solution lies in creating safe ways to release patients earlier, and in ways for patients who are aging in place to heal and get care safely in their homes. That means collecting and analyzing data with a keen eye on taking action when appropriate. Sound familiar? This is next-level connected health. The result is a win-win for all the parties involved in the care experience.

How do all the pieces fit together and work? I sat down with Steve McDonald of ThriveWell to find out.

Steve has a 30-year track record in the healthcare industry, including hospital, ambulatory care, and information technology sectors. He has worked in executive leadership roles at Meditech and Cerner, as well as at Beacon Partners (now KPMG) and Impact Advisors. Steve knows healthcare from a broad perspective, so we asked him a basic question: "Where is home care going?"

"Hospitals now are looking at home care as a viable venue to serve up their own services," Steve says. "One trend is aging in place which more and more seniors are choosing to do. Many are taking advantage of the proliferation of home care devices. It's now very viable to have someone get discharged from the hospital earlier, which is a more cost-effective way to manage their chronic diseases in the comfort of their home."

But how can hospitals let people go home sooner, without hurting health outcomes or incurring legal and financial risk? How can hospitals, for example, be satisfied that patients are recovering at home in a way that equals the care they could have experienced if they had remained inpatients for longer periods of time?

"You need to have information," Steve says. "First, you need the discharge planning notes, and all of the care plans you will need to engage patients when they are discharged from the hospital. That's just one element. You then need to keep your patients engaged from there.

"Wi-Fi capabilities are the foundational technology. At the baseline, you must be connected.

"From a technology perspective, lots of things are built on that connectivity, including video chats, telehealth and remote patient monitoring. Plus, there are many devices that are purposely designed for each chronic condition. Whether a patient has COPD or CHF or diabetes, there is a digital solution for each of them and they all hit your clinician or care provider's radar in a way that recognizes who needs help right now and who is doing fine. But I'm seeing that it's not enough to just throw a device at someone."

WHO WILL PAY FOR ADVANCED AT-HOME CARE?

Steve points out that when it comes to being reimbursed for at-home care, things are changing quickly, and new business models are evolving that allow companies to offer at-home care in ways that make economic sense. Some of the trends Steve cites are:

- **The Centers for Medicare and Medicaid Services** (CMS) have introduced a more liberal reimbursement policy for remote patient monitoring. The net is you now get to go home earlier after hospital stays.

- **Medicaid** has recently adopted parity laws to mandate that telehealth visits be paid at the same price as inpatient visits. Although this varies by state, going home early is the new norm and a growing expectation.

- **New home-care business models** are evolving, some charging a subscription fee for monitoring and connecting you to your clinician and all the specialists servicing your episode of care.

Steve also points out that technology is evolving in ways that provide better remote care.

"Someone has an alert that fires because their blood pressure spikes," Steve cites as an example. "And their phone will ring and there will be a person on the other end who will say, 'Are you OK? Let's find out what caused this. Can we intervene on your behalf to make sure that there's no episode of care that's going to result in an emergency room visit?'

"There are so many devices now that can capture that information at home. And it stands to reason that anyone would prefer to be at home rather than driving to a hospital, trying to find a parking spot, then following the yellow line or the blue line to their doctor's office. It's just a much more affordable approach and a more convenient, more efficient way to be able to manage your chronic diseases." That reduces the friction which often prevents us from getting the care we need.

WHO BENEFITS?

I asked Steve to define the greatest beneficiary of more connected, advanced at-home care. Is it the patient, the provider? Where is this trend evolving?

"The quick answer" Steve told me, "is that both patients and payers benefit quite a bit. With better outcomes, the provider gets reimbursed at a higher rate and makes more money. The patient receives better care, likes the familiarity of being at home, and doesn't have to deal with driving, dealing with traffic, or looking for parking."

Who among the old-school healthcare incumbents could imagine healthcare applying Yelp-scoring concepts where our ratings matter? Are there challenges that could hinder the wider adoption of at-home monitoring and healthcare? I asked Steve.

"I would say there are challenges, depending on the demographic," Steve says. "One is that some seniors don't want to mess with devices. Yet there are ways around that, like passive devices. Maybe it's a sensor under your pillow that can track heart rate or respiration or even a simple ring that your wear like Oura's Sleep Ring and activity trackers.

"The solution can be more of a care-centric model that treats chronic diseases with a combination of devices. And patients, payers, and providers (hospitals) all benefit. Hospitals in risk-based contracts or value-based contracts benefit financially, due to lower costs associated with better health outcomes."

EPISODES OF CARE

An "episode of care" can be defined as a span of time in which a patient receives healthcare to help with a finite health issue. If you break your arm, have a cast put on it, then have the cast removed and undergo a period of physical therapy until you are able to use your arm again normally, that is an episode of care. If you have a rash and go to a dermatologist who gives you a salve to apply and then the rash goes completely away, that is another example of an episode of care.

Yet other episodes of care can last longer, or maybe even never go away. If you know someone who is dealing with diabetes, for example, their episode of care is lifelong.

I mention this concept because considering episodes of care sheds light on the patient experience, including issues like health insurance.

"Aging in place was the beachhead for home care and is a critical piece in managing episodes of care," Steve says, "with a finite time frame to address outcomes of that episode. Additionally, chronic care for COPD, CHF and hypertension are all more effectively maintained with an age-in-place technology solution.

"Yet we have to be realistic and think that there will always be reasons for people to go to hospitals. There are obvious ones, like emergency room visits. There are also triage oncology visits, which involve some really sophisticated diagnostic machinery, like linear accelerators to look at how cancer is growing. Dialysis isn't typically done at home. People are not going to get a hip replacement done there either.

"But regarding that hip replacement, the hospital might say, OK, this person is 58 years old. He's not too fat. He can actually go home and be managed remotely. Or maybe we can send a physical therapist to his house. And that would be incredibly cost-effective.

"A hip replacement typically costs $30,000. That is the average cost, based on actuarial data. Some surgeries will always take place in hospitals. Yet if the patient starts recuperating at home sooner, the cost could be reduced to $21,000. And that care can still hit all the metrics from a quality perspective."

To provide that care, we need to be asking, what kind of care can we provide remotely? Steve foresees a world where smart technologies will appear more and more in home settings.

"We're already seeing smart homes that shut off lights and monitor what is in your fridge and know when it is time to order milk," Steve notes. "From a wellness perspective, a lot of digital health investment is going into wellness."

The result will be lower-cost, better healthcare in a growing number of situations, and conditions. "That's why we're called ThriveWell," Steve adds.

No question about it, things are improving across the board in healthcare, thanks to a combination of technology, compassion, and smart thinking—in whatever combination and alchemy. Thanks to some very smart individuals and their companies, we are surely entering a brave new world of healthcare—one where receiving hospital level care at home is the new normal.

If homecare is indeed the next big thing, then let your mind wander to how Anthem's Sydney platform fits into the equation. I know Sydney was designed from the ground up to be a member benefit for Anthem health plan members, but you can't help but think about how versatile a tool this has become and how that might have a broader impact for us as consumers.

MEET RAJEEV RONANKI OF ANTHEM, INC.

If you spend any time at all with Rajeev Ronanki, you quickly realize that there is probably nobody else in healthcare who knows as much about the realities of how AI can be used to improve patient experiences and outcomes.

Rajeev serves as senior vice president and chief digital officer at Anthem, Inc., where he oversees the vision, strategy, and execution of Anthem's digital, AI, and exponential technology portfolios to move Anthem to become a true AI-first enterprise. In addition, he oversees innovation and modernization, and with his team, drives enterprise data strategies. Before Anthem, Rajeev started and led Deloitte's Life Sciences and Healthcare Advanced Analytics, AI, and Innovation practice. He was also instrumental in shaping Deloitte's blockchain and cryptocurrency solutions and authored pieces on various exponential technology topics. Rajeev also led Deloitte's partnership with Singularity University and start-ups that included doc.AI, OpenAI and MIT Media Lab's MedRec.

Sydney is Anthem's remarkable, AI-driven engagement app that Rajeev was instrumental in developing. Virtually every healthcare company has an app of some kind, but you don't have to spend more than a minute or two on Sydney to see that it is different in the degree of friendliness and functionality that it brings to our smartphones.

Anthem's website states that the Sydney app is simple, smart, and personal. And after a minute or two, you see that is certainly true. I should know. I am not only a big fan, I am a big user.

What can Sydney do?

- **Find care and check costs:** It's easy to search for doctors, dentists, hospitals, labs, and other providers in your plan. You can search by name, location, or the type of care you are seeking. You can even filter by gender or languages spoken, then check costs before you go. This helps you find what's best for you, and you gain an advantage in knowing what to expect before you go in for your visit.

- **See all your benefits**: Sydney shows you essential information at a glance, whether that's an overview of your plan, health reminders or suggestions for wellness programs. You can also find your deductible, copay and share of costs. It is all integrated so there is never any doubt about what is covered, how much is in your health savings account (HSA) and what your out-of-pocket expense will be.

- **Sync with your fitness tracker**: Sydney makes it easy to stay connected to your health. You can easily sync your devices to your fitness trackers and set custom reminders to help you reach your goals. This gives Anthem a more holistic and longitudinal view of who you are and what you do. Knowing your history is an important precursor to knowing how to best help you.

- **Use the interactive chat feature to get answers quickly:** Just type your questions in the app and get the info you need quickly. Plus, Sydney can suggest resources to help you understand your benefits, improve your health, and save money. In the COVID era, this has become an essential feature that addresses all of our needs.

- **View and use digital ID cards:** You can always have your most current ID card handy. And you can use it just like a paper one when you visit the doctor or dentist, pay for care and more. Soon, your HSA debit card will be integrated, meaning you shop for your healthcare needs, know what portions will be covered and pay from your HSA all from one application.

- **View claims:** Check medical, dental and vision claims in one click. That means you can spend more time focused on your health and less on managing your health benefits.

- **Check My Family Health Records (myFHR):** myFHR gives you easy access to your health data, including health history and electronic medical records, all in one place. Availability is based on your Anthem plan.

What makes Sydney different is that, thanks to seamless and invisible AI, it's all simple and intuitive. I have come to think of it as a curated experience where best-of-breed solutions are at my fingertips. Sydney knows my history and what is important to me.

"Pre-pandemic, Sydney was essentially designed as a one-stop shop for all things service-related for Anthem," Rajeev explains. "The idea was to create a simple easy-to-use experience that would allow users to resolve all the issues that would ordinarily be handled on a phone call to customer service. Initially, finding care was the function that it was used for most often. You could also follow up on a claim, make a payment, or do anything you would typically do on a call. Only instead of being placed on hold, you were driving the content with your inquiries at your own pace.

"And then the pandemic hit, and we were looking at ways in which we could bring care options to our members who otherwise would not have access to care. In a matter of a few weeks, we saw a wider range of digital and virtual care options that could be made available in Sydney.

"That was rolled out last April, and we had over 200,000 people that were able to triage symptoms and do preliminary research on symptoms they might be experiencing. Several million people used text, video, and virtual visits. The horse had left the barn so to speak and Sydney's mission evolved overnight. A worldwide healthcare crisis can do that.

"So there was a transition. It started with customer service, but it was always on our roadmap to deliver actual care via Sydney. During the pandemic, we accelerated that and integrated digital and virtual primary care, and we've made that available to all of our members. They used Sydney to find vaccination sites, track when vaccinations were actually being administered, and schedule appointments. Those resulting patient records could be used by the appropriate vaccine passport providers, as a way of validating that people actually got their vaccinations. And the data can be used to analyze and understand trends and patterns in Covid care both at the micro and macro level."

When I interviewed Rajeev two years ago for my first book *The Digital Health Revolution,* Sydney was really more of a vision. Now, Rajeev tells me that about 20 million Anthem members are using Sydney which certainly answers initial questions about scaling. During the pandemic, Sydney was used about 11 million times, on computers, tablets, and smartphones.

GOODBYE TO LIVE CARE?

Clearly, Anthem is embracing digital technologies. But does that mean that live care experiences are about to go away?

I asked Rajeev.

"I think maybe we define telehealth too narrowly," Rajeev told me, then he went on to explain, "there was definitely a spike in usage of specialized telehealth networks. We define digital care as care that does not require a human at the other end, whether that is a nurse, a doctor, a caregiver or care manager. There are things that we could do that are automated, based on our data. One goal is for users to be able to understand what is best for them to do next, based on our insights.

"Let's say that our data indicates that the next best step for a member is to see a doctor. We want to be able to provide multiple options for doing just that. The user, for example, can either text or email a doctor, which can lead to an in-person appointment, or a video consultation. But the user would be able to seamlessly bridge into that.

"There are times when a physical service is needed. Maybe the patient needs to have blood drawn. So, how do we get that done for Anthem members? Do we have our member go to a local lab somewhere? Do we send someone to his or her home? We want to integrate that on Sydney. We have both ways of doing it.

"If an in-person service is required, we want to keep that continuum flowing seamlessly; we can schedule an appointment, get the procedure taken care of, and then follow up with digital virtual remote monitoring care so that that loop continues to be seamless and continuous between digital, virtual and physical. And then, from a member's perspective, it's all seamless. If that care needs to be rendered at home, so be it. If it can be done virtually—terrific. If it requires an in-person visit because lab work is required—not a problem.

"That seamless experience is something that's hard to find on many services, where experiences are siloed. You can download an app and track your symptoms, but that really doesn't go anywhere or connect to all that you need to really be a seamless experience. You can have a telehealth consultation, or you could get a discount pharmacy card somewhere and get your prescriptions mailed to your home by connecting to your prescriber. But there is no larger awareness of what is happening with your health, no context or medical history. Do you have allergies? Have you experienced side effects after using a medication? That information might not be captured.

"If none of that is integrated, then everyone's operating sort of in the blind. But we're connecting all the dots, so that on our platforms, the data breadcrumbs carry forward seamlessly and we're able to provide insights at each interaction." For homecare to ever be an accepted norm, this is essential.

AI AND INDIVIDUATION

Rajeev and his team have worked hard to have AI provide an experience in which each member's search for care solutions is different—highly individuated.

"My search could be different from yours," Rajeev says. "Each search should be tailored to our unique set of fingerprints, our health history. And that results in a very curated sort of presentation of network options or doctors' choices, which is no different than how Netflix matches up users with content.

"We match up our users with appropriate providers, based on hundreds of attributes that have been uniquely curated. So that's a far richer experience than what people will discover on popular internet apps that provide information on health.

"The information those internet apps give is not always connected—it's purely informational. Again, nothing is connected to a user's individual data. If you need an appointment, that online page is not going to schedule one for you. Your health history will not be there. If you have an in-person appointment with a care provider you have never seen before, you are going to have to provide information on your medical history and your medications all over again. When we talk about reducing the friction associated with getting the care we need, this is always at the top of everyone's list of pet peeves. How many times do I have to provide my doctors with the same information? What the heck are they doing with my data if they have to ask me for it every time I step through their front door?

"For Anthem members who use Sydney, all those assets are available at their fingertips now. Let me say, Sydney is not available in every market for every provider, because we're still in the process of connecting all the providers into our platform. We are making that universally available, but it's very much a work in progress."

AI AND THE DEMOCRATIZATION OF HEALTHCARE

Over the years, I have often heard it said that your zip code can serve as a better predictor of your long-term health than your genetics. And we now know just how true that is. Who suffered the poorest health outcomes during Covid-19, for example? The people who lived in the least wealthy locales in America. They had the poorest access to good food and often, the poorest access to hospitals and other healthcare providers.

AI, which most people think of as a way of making computers more communicative and smarter, can really level the playing field in that situation. The reach and availability of AI-enhanced apps is growing day by day, with the increasing numbers of smartphones in use in inner cities, in America's rural regions—everywhere.

"AI is here to stay," says Rajeev. "It's already part and parcel of every industry, or it will be in the near future. It's something that every industry is going to have to learn to adopt and apply to optimize their businesses. Healthcare is no different. In fact, healthcare is the top industry where AI has the greatest potential and benefit."

ETHICAL CONSIDERATIONS

"There absolutely is a risk in the expanded ability of our models and algorithms," Rajeev says. "I think there's bias, there are ethics to consider. And all these things have to be very carefully thought through while implementing and scaling IT programs, because the fact of the matter is that bias and inequities exist in the healthcare system today. We need to make sure that we are not furthering those biases.

"As we touched upon earlier, your zip code can greatly influence your health outcomes, perhaps even more than your genetics. So if that's the case, there is a danger of turning what is perhaps a non-scalable bias in humans into something that's infinitely scalable. There is a risk of perpetuating the normal checks and balances of decision-making and making them more dangerous when applied at a machine scale.

"So to mitigate that, we have to be very consciously designing for governance and testing for data quality. We need to be building checks and balances into the algorithms to account for all the things you referenced, Kevin. At Anthem we have a robust program around responsibility, which includes governance, ethics, bias.

"We routinely check our work from an independent lens to ask, 'While we are solving one problem, are we doing something that will create or perpetuate another problem?' We look for data quality issues, we look for holes in the way most algorithms are developed and take every practical step we can to mitigate any bias. We also need solutions around the completeness of data sets, because if only certain kinds of data are considered, or considered incompletely—demographics, for example, or certain geographies—then inherently the knowledge base is not accurate. It might not be representative of the entire population.

"But then, if that's the case, how do we get the healthcare data for the rest of the population if they're never in the system? So I think there have to be more collective industry efforts to create a broader dataset and have a lot of rigor in making sure that that data is complete, has integrity, and represents the entirety of population to make sure that we're using complete data to build the ground floor of a scaling area, if you will."

EARNING TRUST

I have noticed that trust or lack thereof can be the greatest enabler of any new technology. In healthcare, if end-users do not trust a provider or an app to protect their data, for example, then that solutions provider will simply not succeed. I am not surprised that Rajeev, who with his team is introducing a new way of interacting with consumers and their data, also views trust as a prerequisite for success.

"Trust is absolutely foundational to all of this," Rajeev says. "So Anthem is presenting options and engaging our users and members in highly considered and careful ways. We can't reach the entire spectrum of our population if they don't trust what we're serving up. And if they don't believe we're acting in their best interests, we're not going to get the adoption that we need to get. Said a different way, we need to be solving real world healthcare problems and adding value in a near real time environment.

"Trust starts with the premise that consumers should own their own healthcare data. From a practical perspective, that means that everyone in the system should make it as easy as possible to let consumers have access to their data in a way that's easy and affordable and simple to navigate.

"If we start there and say to consumers, `You're in charge of your own data, you tell us how you want to use it. We, of course, would like the privilege of using that data to improve our algorithm and insights. But if you'd rather have us not use it, we'll find other ways to find a solution.' That is easier said than done, and I think every industry struggles with it.

"I think big tech has not done us any favors with the way that they've approached the problem and we've got to overcome that. You think along the lines of Facebook and Google during the election process, and it sends a chill up your spine. But unless we overcome that, I believe our future, where our healthcare experiences are very much like a retail experience, is going to be hard to pull off at scale."

RAJEEV SUMS IT UP

"At the end of the day, it's all about simplifying. So between your life and your watch and your phone and all the other sensors and all the data that you're probably inundated with, how do you simplify it and engage just with the minimal amount of information that's necessary to create the optimal outcome?

"For Anthem, that is what it comes down to—how do you create that human-centered, design-led approach to presenting all of this information in a way that's meaningful and actionable? And how do we address the needs of a family of four that's worried about homework, jobs, and commutes and not only health maintenance and care? We need a really simple, simplified way to engage. We need to profoundly simplify the experience. Then we can serve up the things at the right moment to create the right outcome and intervention."

Sounds a lot like meeting people where they are. They live in the real world, not the healthcare world and increasingly, that means being able to coordinate their care needs from home.

To add value in the real world, all of these devices, apps, and platforms need to be solving real world healthcare problems and meeting us where we are. We can and should be able to govern who can see and use our health data. Trust will always be key and being able to take action on our health data to receive an immediate benefit will be the expectation. You aren't healthy the day after you quit smoking just like you don't get fat by eating one piece of cake. Well, my wife might argue that last point, but you get the idea. Everyone wants a quick fix, but devices, apps and policy don't make us healthy—we do.

So plug in and get connected. Healthcare has been innovating. It is time to catch up. All you need is your smartphone.

IN CLOSING, LET'S HEAR AGAIN
FROM SENATOR BILL FRIST

Because I was born and raised in Vermont, my pulse quickens when a thought leader draws lessons learned from rural markets when identifying larger trends and making predictions. Let's turn again to Senator Bill Frist, a native of Tennessee, who leans in and doesn't shy from the most vexing of healthcare delivery challenges.

"Kevin," Senator Frist told me, "It's a broader question than about where you personally started out. Rural healthcare is something that nobody has been able to address. In rural areas, there is a higher burden of disease, more obesity, more opioid use, more hypertension, higher infant mortality and higher overall mortality.

"You have to remember, about 60% of our nation's population resides in rural communities. That represents a unique challenge. In rural areas there is less access to primary care. There are fewer specialists, less access to nurses and tertiary or secondary hospitals.

"Tennessee has 49 hospitals today. Eleven have gone out of business in the last 10 years. Of the 49 rural hospitals we have today, 25 are at risk for closure. And 23 of those are at *immediate* risk for closure. So, we have a higher burden of disease paired with a very low supply. The trends are all going in the wrong direction with closure of care. That problem is just going to get worse.

"Why? Because of a lack of cultural sensitivity. I put that number one, and that's where everybody else out there will continue to fail because they say, 'I've got the technology and I'll throw it at the problem.' But that's not going to do it. We need cultural sensitivity.

"In general, we've got the building blocks in the community to be culturally sensitive. You have some primary care-providers and urgent care centers that are trying to focus on rural healthcare. Plus, you have independent pharmacies which have been underutilized until now.

"Capturing the tailwind of a fee-for-service system, moving to value-based care, you will find people starting to focus on outcomes instead of individual services being delivered in a chaotic and unconnected way.

"But things can always get better, and it is really not that hard. That said, nobody has actually been able to do it just yet."

How will it happen? When I spoke with Senator Frist, he was just about to announce the debut of a company called Main Street Health and that could be a predictor of the kind of change we are about to see happen in rural markets.

"It will be a culturally sensitive organization from day one," Senator Frist says, and "it will be able to integrate the independent pharmacies, the urgent care centers and the local doctors and nurses in a way that's built around that true value-based care.

"Other people have tried, and we know the health plans and payers want it. They are responsible for covering the cost of caring for those patients, but they are just not delivering. Some are simply too big to innovate. They have too many other responsibilities that they regard as bigger, louder voices. They can't focus on vulnerable populations in rural areas especially."

But when the changes that Senator Frist envisions happen, what will they look like from a consumer's perspective?

"In a rural community of 3,000 people, when someone wakes up in the middle of the night and needs care, all they can do is go to a hospital. Hopefully, there is a hospital nearby. But the goal of innovative companies will increasingly be to offer access to real physicians who will be working with nurses.

"That's the way it is. Nurses do a better job than a lot of doctors with 24/7 access – say, in a community that's four hours from Nashville or Memphis, where a hospital can be three or four counties away. Digital health technologies can connect people to care wherever they live, likely from nurse practitioners.

"That sort of alignment just hasn't been done before. Obviously, we'll use telemedicine and virtual care. We have the advantage now that a lot of the specialists are used to doing that. They weren't, pre-Covid, but now they are. And that's going to make our job a lot easier."

AFTERWORD
A DAY IN THE LIFE

Woke up, fell out of bed
Dragged the comb across my head
Found my way downstairs and drank a cup
And looking up, I noticed I was late
Found my coat and grabbed by hat
Made the bus in seconds' flat
—,The Beatles
"A Day in The Life"

How many of us can relate? Maybe the Covid version should be "Made the Zoom in seconds flat"? The point is, we are all creatures of habit and mine have taken a turn toward the healthy. I haven't always been like this. In my first book, I told the story of growing up in rural Vermont, how we were constantly on the go—riding bikes, playing ball, fishing, swimming and eating what we grew, or nature provided. Somewhere along the way, life came at me hard and fast. There were jobs with unbearable everyday train commutes and then endless amounts of air travel. I learned early on that if you traveled, you made more money, and we were a single income household, so I signed up. Then came the children and they needed to be nurtured, fed, clothed and loved. My routines changed from being active and constantly on the go, to long daily commutes capped by family TV shows at night with barely any time for decompression time between work and family. I used to joke that we will sleep when we die and that probably almost happened. Now, the question I ask myself is why did I wait so long to learn how to rest? We all need it, and we all perform better when there is balance in our lives.

One of my earliest and most notable mentors was Lucia Hicks

Williams, who was my manager at Sybase. She once told me that it is a myth that people don't like change. Who wouldn't be excited about a new home, new car or a new job? It is the transition we struggle with. Maybe the new home has termites and needs electrical work. The new car gets lousy gas mileage, and you feel every bump in the road. The new job comes with an incredibly expensive commute. And yet, we muscle through it all until these new routines become baked into our daily cadence and accepted as normal. Before long, we can't imagine it any other way. It is human nature to thrill to the concept of change and then struggle with the associated transitions that come with it. Those who learn how to manage change are destined to thrive. These are your innovators. They can create structure from ambiguity and have confidence in their ability to navigate life's uncertainties. They also fully understand that change, we must. Leveraging behavioral principles is key to sustaining any meaningful or sustainable change in lifestyle. What is your agent of change? I like gizmos, gadgets and content that helps me understand why doing something different isn't just a good idea, it is essential.

I am happy to say that much of what I described in the afterword in my first book, *The Digital Health Revolution,* is still very much a part of my life. I still step on my scale every morning; I still take a moment to check my blood pressure and share that data to platforms that help me make sense of how everyday lifestyle choices affect my health in a measurable way. I have even added a few new routines. On my way to the kitchen before pouring a cup and reading my morning brief, I exhale into my Lumen. It helps me calibrate my diet to my daily activities and provides important recommendations on what I need to eat that day to optimize my calorie burn. Improved metabolism has put me on the course of better weight management. Today, breakfast is sliced fresh fruit, berries and a tall glass of water. Tomorrow's recommendation may mean adding a protein like eggs or smoked salmon. Lumen is listening to my body and helping me calibrate my diet. To help get a better longitudinal view, I log what I eat in Noom, another new habit I have developed. I am still a new user of Noom and truthfully this one is not yet fully baked into my normal routines but hey, I am trying! I find that when my diet is good, I can't wait to post and track and when my sweet tooth kicks in, well, not so much. Noom tells me this is normal and helps me power through to get a more consistent view of what I tend to eat and when I fall off stride.

To be fair, nothing has stressed my new daily "normal" like Covid. The gym was closed for nearly a year and my scale reminded me of the effects of those missed activities. Walking is great but not nearly enough. At my age, the occasional massage and steam room helps keep my muscles relaxed and flexible. Like any athlete, my body craves a variety of workouts and the precision and focus required by sports like basketball, tennis and golf helps me scratch that itch. When I am doing these activities, my body and mind seem to heal. Nothing else matters when I am in the zone. Remove that and well, you have transition issues. Covid easily contributed an additional 15-20 pounds, so I am diving back into my old routines—the ones that helped me get fit in the first place. Only now, I have a lot more help. My fitness instructor monitors the workouts I share with her, and she makes timely suggestions for how to clear plateaus that sometimes stymy me. EatFitGo delivers prepared meals and that makes eating sensible fun and easy. I would be remiss if I didn't also say EatFitGo is tasty. When I check in for my annual physical with One Medical, they get a year's worth of data on a dashboard view. Together, we are working through why there are periods when blood pressure, cholesterol and weight spiral in the wrong direction. Understanding cause and effect is critical. The anniversary of my father and my brother passing has always challenged me. One Medical helps me understand that these psychological triggers can send me off in a bad direction. Every fall, I brace for life's reminder that we all have an expiration tag and two loved ones whom I still dearly miss are no longer here. That can take a toll on anyone. We are all human. I never realized that my biometrics going out of whack every winter was tied to anything. I used to joke it was my winter weight and normalized that we all get it. Truth is, it typically kicked off an extended period of inactivity that cratered my energy and sent my weight and blood pressure in the wrong direction.

To help stay grounded and centered, I like to garden, so every day I wander out into the berry patch and vegetable garden to water and give them some love. It is relaxing and it gives me an activity to do with my 85-year-old mother-in-law who truthfully gets most of the credit for our backyard looking so nice. Together, we collaborate on what to plant and where it goes. Her golden rule? Water the roots! (Audrey is always right!)

Our garden is now producing raspberries, blackberries, blueberries and strawberries. The apple orchard provides us with MacIntosh, Empire, Pink Lady, Honeycrisp and Empire apples. The citrus grove is now cranking out more mandarins, grapefruits, lemons, limes and oranges than we can possibly eat. When life gives you oranges and lemons—you juice! We have since added a new avocado tree, a mango tree, a couple of bananas and a papaya tree. California sunshine is great for tropical planting and next year we are looking to add pomegranates and a chocolate plant. The gardening relaxes me, but the fruits and berries are what bring my nephews and nieces outside on our treasure hunts. My wife is all about the herbs, peppers, rhubarb and tomatoes. I go into withdrawal whenever I leave them alone for too long. I worry they will atrophy. One pro tip I have learned is that from deer to raccoons and skunks, all varmints seem to detest mint and peppermint, so I always surround my garden with them to keep out the critters. Now, if I could only do something about those birds! These routines are now baked into my daily schedule.

I am up at sunrise to get a good jump on my day and gardening time is something I look forward to doing.

One routine I remain faithful to no matter the weather or time of year is my daily walk with my wife Beth and our dog Chuey. This is our time. We decompress, we vent, we let go... We are there for one another and this is our reminder of what is truly important in life—our family. Growing up in one of the most dilapidated corners of New England, it was never a guarantee that one day we would be so blessed. There are many reasons to give thanks. Our childhood experiences help shape who we are, but they don't fully define us. You have a chance every day to exemplify what really matters in life. For me that is health, happiness and family. They are all intertwined. When I am taking care of myself, I can be there for others. When I do for others, they feel inspired to do for me. We are better together in my household.

I have come to appreciate that who we are is comprised as much of how we feel as our biometrics like weight and blood pressure. What we do and how we eat are fundamental pillars to getting and staying healthy. If we can teach that to children as they are growing up and then reinforce that at school and then later at work, we are taking a massive step toward lowering the cost of healthcare in America. There is no magic policy wand we can wave to achieve good health. Diabetes doesn't care if you are on a public or private healthcare system. How we live our lives matters. We all have a participative role to play.

EXPERT CONTRIBUTORS

Oron Afek

Oron Afek is the co-founder and CEO of Vim (www.getvim.com) a company that improves network performance and enhances its member experience. The inspiration behind Vim is to provide solutions to healthcare customers wherever they are—online, in doctors' offices, or in hospitals or other care facilities. The philosophy is to improve customers' lives by making healthcare work better.

Prior to Vim, Oron started a telecommunication-focused startup company which was acquired by a large mobile operator, as well as a gaming company in Tel Aviv, Israel. Oron also started and managed a Barcelona-based REIT. Prior to his commercial career, Oron served in the Israeli special forces.

Austin Beutner

Austin Beutner is a civic leader and public servant who has worked for the last decade to make Los Angeles a stronger community. Mr. Beutner was appointed superintendent of Los Angeles Unified School District (https://achieve.lausd.net), the nation's second largest, in May 2018. Under his leadership, Los Angeles Unified has led the nation in responding to the crisis in public schools created by Covid-19. The school district has provided 128 million meals along with 30 million items of needed supplies to the communities it serves, made sure all students have a computer and free internet access to remain connected with their school community, created student-centered learning shows which are being used by PBS affiliates and school districts in 30 states, and is providing Covid-19 tests to students and staff at schools with the support of a consortium including world-class research universities, bio-tech testing companies, health insurers, a technology giant and a national medical center. Mr. Beutner has served as first deputy mayor of Los Angeles, publisher and CEO of the *Los Angeles Times* and *San Diego Union Tribune* and co-chair of the Los Angeles 2020 Commission and the LA Unified Advisory Task Force.

He holds a degree in economics from Dartmouth College, and has taught courses in ethics, leadership and effective government at Harvard Business School, University of Southern California Price School of Public Policy, the UCLA Anderson School of Management, and California State University Northridge. He founded Vision to Learn, a non-profit organization that has provided free eye exams and glasses to more than 250,000 children at schools in low-income communities across the country.

Stevon Cook

In 2016, Stevon Cook was elected to the San Francisco Board of Education after receiving more than 150,00 votes. He served as president of the board of education in 2018 and 2019. During his tenure, he passed nationally recognized policies on K-12 black studies, reforming school assignment and expanding access to college courses for all students.

Stevon is a fourth generation San Franciscan and alumnus of Thurgood Marshall High School in Bayview-Hunters Point. During his undergraduate years at Williams College, he became active in business and a leader in a community service organization called the Griffin's Society. Upon graduating with a degree in American Studies, he returned to San Francisco to serve in the first graduating class of the Mayor's City Hall Fellows program.

Prior to his election, Stevon served as CEO of Mission Bit, where he created community initiatives with a number of public and private entities such as the San Francisco mayor's Office of Economic Development, Golden State Warriors, Adobe, Salesforce and school districts across the bay area. The organization has grown to serve over 10,000 students and continues to make tremendous impact after his departure in May 2019. Stevon continues to provide support to elected officials across the country in the areas of educational strategy and policy.

Ray Costantini

Ray Costantini, MD, is co-founder and CEO of Bright.md (www.bright.md). Founded in 2012, Bright.md's SmartExam platform serves as a "virtual physician assistant" for primary care providers, gathering information from patients who submit clinical surveys, select pharmacies, and enter insurance information. The company states that it is "the digital thread that ties care offerings together."

Ray is a pioneering healthcare executive, an innovative physician, and a seasoned entrepreneur who is passionate about making healthcare better. Prior to founding Bright.md, he led the design, build, deployment, and operations of three groundbreaking telehealth and digital health products at Providence Health and Services, one of the largest health systems in the country. He also previously founded three successful companies and is a national speaker on healthcare innovation, telehealth, and patient engagement.

Brad Fluegel

Brad Fluegel currently advises healthcare organizations, entrepreneurs, private equity, and other participants in healthcare. He recently retired from being the senior vice president and chief strategy officer at Walgreens (www.walgreens.com). Brad now serves on the board of directors at Metropolitan Jewish Health System in New York City, Performant Financial Corporation, Fitbit, Premera Blue Cross and Alight Solutions.

Brad earned a master's degree in public policy from Harvard University's Kennedy School of Government and a Bachelor of Arts in business administration from the University of Washington. He also serves as a lecturer at the University of Pennsylvania's Wharton School of Business.

Senator William Frist

Senator William Frist, MD, is a nationally-acclaimed heart and lung transplant surgeon, former U.S. Senate Majority Leader, founding partner of Frist Cressey Ventures and chairman of the Executives Council of the health service investment firm Cressey & Company. He is actively engaged in the business, medical, humanitarian, and philanthropic communities.

Senator Frist annually has led medical mission trips to Africa and Haiti, and emergency response teams to disasters around the globe, including to Sri Lanka after the Indian Ocean tsunami, Bangladesh, Sudan, New Orleans after Katrina, Haiti after the earthquake, and the Horn of Africa. He is chairman of both Hope Through Healing Hands, which focuses on maternal and child health and global poverty, and SCORE, a statewide collaborative education reform organization that has helped propel Tennessee to prominence as a K12 education reform state.

Bob Gold

Bob Gold is founder, CEO, and chief behavioral technologist at GoMo Health (www.gomohealth.com), an innovative New Jersey-based company that is a leader in designing, implementing, and marketing award-winning, personalized patient engagement solutions that support the continuum of care. Bob and his team have developed what they call Behavioral Rx, which they describe as a scalable and cost-effective way that companies can use to engage with end-users that enables better self-management, healthy decisions, and improved outcomes.

Bob is one of the world's leading behavioral technologists with more than 20 years applied research and development in the behavioral and cognitive science of human motivation, activation and resiliency; with a specialty in the human and social factors of individualized precision health digital therapies leading to increased activation of patients and clinicians in underserved vulnerable communities, both urban and rural.

Sheila Hamilton

Sheila Hamilton is the CEO of Beyond Well Solutions (www.beyondwellsolutions.com). Her company provides a mental health solution for employers who want to engage employees in better behavioral health and wellness.

Sheila is a five-time Emmy-winning mental health journalist, and the author of *All the Things We Never Knew: Chasing the Chaos of Mental Illness*. Among the many awards she has won are the Ron Schmidt Community Service Award and the Judy Cushing Life Award for her advocacy for people with mental illness. She hosts the podcast *Beyond Well with Sheila Hamilton*.

Ann Mond Johnson

Ann Mond Johnson joined the American Telemedicine Association (ATA) as CEO in 2018. Her experience includes building, launching and leading client-driven companies that have been innovators in healthcare technology and data to support consumers using healthcare.

Peter V. Lee

Peter V. Lee is the first executive director for California's health benefit exchange, Covered California (www. hbex.ca.gov). Having been confirmed unanimously by the exchange board in 2011, he oversees the planning, development, ongoing administration and evaluation of Covered California and its efforts to improve the affordability and accessibility of quality healthcare for Californians.

Prior to his current role as executive director of Covered California, Peter served as the deputy director for the Center for Medicare and Medicaid Innovation at the Centers for Medicare and Medicaid Services (CMS) in Washington, D.C., where he led initiatives to identify, test and support new models of care in Medicare and Medicaid—resulting in higher quality care while reducing costs.

Previously Peter was the Director of Delivery System Reform for the Office of Health Reform for the U.S. Department of Health and Human Services, where he coordinated delivery reform efforts for Secretary Kathleen Sebelius and assisted in the preparation of the National Quality Strategy. Before joining the Obama administration, Peter served from 2000-2008 as the CEO and executive Director for National Health Policy of the Pacific Business Group on Health (PBGH), one of the leading coalitions of private and public purchasers in the nation. Peter also served as the executive director of the Center for Healthcare Rights, a consumer advocacy organization based in Los Angeles from 1995-2000, and was the former Director of Programs for the National AIDS Network.

Prior to his work in public service, Peter was a practicing attorney in Los Angeles. A native Californian, Peter holds a Juris Doctorate from the University of Southern California and a Bachelor of Arts from the University of California, Berkeley.

Alex Lenox-Miller

Alex Lenox-Miller is a senior analyst with Chilmark Research (www.chilmarkresearch.com), a small analysis and consulting firm in Boston that develops comprehensive studies on a number of healthcare topics. Prior to joining Chilmark, Alex was head of analytics for process improvement at Lahey Health, a Massachusetts-based organization that manages hospitals, physicians, and other health services in north-eastern Massachusetts.

Alex's wife is a nurse, and his mother is a physician. Healthcare is almost literally in Alex's bloodstream.

Steve McDonald

Steve McDonald is Chief Commercial Officer at ThriveWell. Steve joined ThriveWell Tech with a 30-year track record in the healthcare industry including hospital, ambulatory care and information technology sectors. He worked in executive leadership roles at Meditech and Cerner, as well as at Beacon Partners (now KPMG) and Impact Advisors. His career reflects solid achievements and leadership in new business development, client management, resource and people management, IT project management and IT consulting management.

Abner Mason

Abner Mason is the founder and CEO of ConsejoSano (www.ConsejoSano.com), the only patient engagement and care navigation solution designed to help clients activate their multicultural patient and member populations to better engage with the healthcare system. ConsejoSano's clients are typically health plans and provider groups serving Medicaid and Medicare Advantage members and patient populations.

Before creating ConsejoSano, Abner was founder and CEO for the Workplace Wellness Council of Mexico, now the leading corporate wellness company in Mexico. From 2003-2008, he was founder and executive director of AIDS Responsibility Project, driving the creation of CONAES and JaBCHA, the first business councils on HIV/AIDS in Mexico and Jamaica. Abner previously served as chairman of the International Committee and member of the Presidential Advisory Council on HIV/AIDS (PACHA), appointed by President Bush in 2002. He spent ten years in the Massachusetts state government, including roles as Chief Policy Advisor to Massachusetts Governors Paul Cellucci and Jane Swift, Governor Cellucci's Undersecretary of Transportation, and Deputy General Manager of the Massachusetts Transit Authority. Before joining state government, Abner worked as an associate consultant for Bain & Company. In 2018, he founded HealthTech 4 Medicaid (HT4M), a non-profit coalition of health-tech leaders collaborating to create technology for Medicaid programs. Additionally, he is a founding council member of United States of Care, a nonprofit centered on improving healthcare access developed by former Medicare/Medicaid administrator Andy Slavitt. Abner is a graduate of Harvard.

Giovanni Monti

Giovanni Monti, senior vice president and director of Healthcare Innovation for Walgreens Boots Alliance (www.walgreens.com), the first global pharmacy-led health and wellbeing enterprise. Prior to creating and leading the HIP, Giovanni was the director of corporate development and mergers and acquisitions at WBA, using his strong expertise in corporate development, M&A, and management consulting. He holds a degree in economic and social sciences from Bocconi University, Milan, an MBA from Columbia Business School and an MIA (master of international affairs) from the School of International and Public Affairs at Columbia University.

Kevin Mullin

Kevin Mullin is chair of the Green Mountain Care Board (gmcboard.vermont.gov). He is tasked with directing the board's charge of curbing healthcare cost growth and reforming the way healthcare is provided to Vermonters.

Kevin spent the majority of his career as a small business owner. He is a graduate of Castleton University with a degree in finance and has taught at the Community College of Vermont and served on numerous community and professional boards. He served 19 years in the Vermont legislature including four years in the House and fifteen years in the Senate, where he served on committees including as chair of the Senate Education and Senate Economic Development, Housing, and General Affairs Committees. As a member of the Senate Health and Welfare Committee, he helped to write both Catamount Health and Green Mountain Care legislation. He has a deep commitment to improving the lives of Vermonters by improving healthcare quality and controlling healthcare spending.

Torben Nielsen

Torben Nielsen is CEO of ZoomCare (www.zoom-care.com), a rapidly growing innovator in on-demand retail and virtual healthcare in six major markets (Seattle, Portland, Eugene, Boise, Boulder, Denver). With 60+ neighborhood clinics and a comprehensive telehealth offering (chat, phone, video), ZoomCare provides same-day primary care, urgent care, specialty care and emergency care to over 300,000 patients a year.

Torben has 20+ years of broad business experience, ranging from nimble start-ups to household brand names such as LEGO, XEROX, and BlueCross BlueShield. His leadership landed ZoomCare among the top ten most admired healthcare companies in Oregon and southwest Washington in 2020, and he was recognized by the *Portland Business Journal* and its readership as one of ten "Executive of the Year" honorees in 2021. He is a co-founder of HealthSparq—the second-fastest-growing digital health company in the U.S. in 2016—and has shepherded innovative, digital healthcare solutions over the past 15 years.

Before entering healthcare, Torben managed marketing, online, retail, and product teams at technology and consumer companies. His work and leadership have been recognized in case studies performed by leading research institutions, including Forrester Research, PwC, and the Advisory Board. Torben has an MBA from Oregon State University and graduated from the Aarhus School of Business in Denmark with an MA in English.

David Pastrana

David Pastrana is the chief executive officer for Jenny Craig. He is a transformational business leader internationally known for his keen acumen in product development and merchandising, operational optimization and brand innovation. David brings more than 15 years of experience in president and C-Level roles, leading global multi-billion-dollar consumer retailers and top industry brands through enterprise and digital transformations to deliver business growth.

David was born and raised in Madrid, where he and his community practiced what he calls a Mediterranean diet. He holds an undergraduate degree in mechanical engineering from Universidad Carlos III de Madrid and a master of business administration, retail and consumer goods, from INSEAD, Fontainebleau, France.

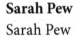

Sarah Pew

Sarah Pew is GM, SVP at W3LL, where she leads the entire business unit. Her top priorities include developing and implementing a strategic vision for W3LL and identifying key investment opportunities. In addition, she monitors healthcare trends, helps maintain a strong company culture, and oversees company communication strategies.

Tom Rifai

Tom Rifai, MD, is the inventor of the "5 Keys to Optimal Wellness" and America's flexitarian lifestyle leader. He is the founder of Reality Meets Science (www.realitymeetsscience.com), a forward-thinking, customer-journey focused digital wellness company.

Tom helps clients and patients achieve metabolic health, food behavior modification and transformational lifestyle change. He has accumulated over 20,000 hours of clinical and leadership experience directing and designing multidisciplinary intensive lifestyle intervention programs, including Henry Ford Health System, where his 5 Keys lifestyle change system is the gold standard for their metabolic health programs.

Tom is the primary author and online course director of Harvard's "Nutrition and the Metabolic Syndrome" program which integrates his "5 Keys to Optimal Wellness." It is one of Harvard's most popular online Lifestyle Medicine courses, attended by more than 4,000 doctors and other healthcare providers worldwide. Tom has written extensively about those 5 keys and is currently writing a book on what he calls a flexitarian lifestyle that is based on them.

Rajeev Ronanki

Rajeev is senior vice president and chief digital officer at Anthem (www.anthem.com), where he oversees the vision, strategy, and execution of Anthem's digital, artificial intelligence (AI) and exponential technology portfolios to move Anthem to become a true AI-first enterprise. In addition, he oversees innovation and modernization, and with his team, drives enterprise data strategies.

Before Anthem, Rajeev started and led Deloitte's Life Sciences and Healthcare Advanced Analytics, AI, and Innovation practice. He was also instrumental in shaping Deloitte's blockchain and cryptocurrency solutions and authored pieces on various exponential technology topics. Rajeev also led Deloitte's partnership with Singularity University and start-ups that included doc. AI, OpenAI and MIT Media Lab's MedRec.

Harpreet Singh Rai

Harpreet Singh Rai is CEO of Oura (www.ouraring. com), where he helped develop the Oura Sleep Ring, one of the most innovative health wearables on the market today.

Harpreet is a true renaissance man in the world of healthcare. He studied electrical engineering at the University of Michigan and launched his business career with Morgan Stanley's merger and acquisitions group. He then led the technology, media, and telecom portfolio for nine years at Eminence Capital.

Constance Sjoquist

Constance Sjoquist, health transformation analyst, is one of the preeminent thought leaders in the health industry today. For more than 25 years, she has guided companies that have been transforming health through disruptive technologies and forward-thinking business strategies to meet the ever-changing landscape of health and technology.

Most recently, Constance was chief transformation officer at HLTH (www.hlth.com), where she helped create the largest and most important conference for health innovation. As one of the primary architects in shaping the voice and creating the agenda for a new conversation on how to improve health, Constance leveraged her cross-industry insights into a robust platform for market disruption and industry transformation. During her tenure, HLTH grew from just a concept to one of the leading industry events with over 7,500 senior leaders spanning every corner of health—payers, providers, pharma, employers, policy-makers, investors, startups, suppliers, retailers, analysts, and associations—and focused on creating the future of health.

Prior to joining HLTH, Constance was a healthcare research director at Gartner, where she covered digital platforms, health exchanges, consumer personalization and engagement, and payment integrity and fraud, waste, and abuse.

Justin Steinman

As chief medical officer of Definitive Healthcare (www.go.definitivehc.com), Justin is responsible for the strategy, development, and execution of all aspects of marketing for the company, including product marketing, demand generation, corporate marketing, public relations, and corporate communications.

Prior to joining Definitive Healthcare, Justin served as the vice president of commercial product management at Aetna, a CVS Health company. Previously, he served as chief marketing officer at GE Healthcare Digital, and in a variety of sales and marketing roles at Novell.

Justin holds undergraduate degrees in English and history from Dartmouth College, and an MBA from the MIT Sloan School of Management.

Ari Tulla

Ari Tulla is co-founder of Elo Health (www.elo.health), a precision nutrition company with a mission to turn food from a cause of disease into medicine. Before Elo, Ari was the CEO of Quest Analytics, a doctor data management and network analytics company. Before Quest Analytics, Ari was the co-founder and CEO of BetterDoctor, a comprehensive doctor data engine that powers the healthcare market with accurate doctor data.

But Ari took an unusual route to becoming a leader in healthcare. Before moving to the healthcare world, he led Nokia's game and application studios, where he was responsible for creating thousands of mobile apps with over 100 million downloads. Ari has two decades of experience in developing new delightful products and experiences. Ari is an entrepreneur, board member, dad, and rock climber—solving problems that help people live better lives.

D.J. Wilson

D.J. Wilson is CEO of State of Reform (www.stateofreform.com), a nonprofit organization headquartered in Washington state. State of Reform's mission is to bridge the gap between healthcare and public policy, reporting on 15 states and federal health policy.

D.J. earned his undergraduate degree from Gonzaga University and an MA in international economics from Johns Hopkins. Prior to joining State of Reform, D.J. was publisher and CEO of *The Washington State Wire*.

Murray Zucker

Murray Zucker, MD, is the medical director at Happify Health (www.happifyhealth.com). As a psychiatrist with a background in academia, large group practice, and health plan clinical executive leadership, he brings expertise in medical behavioral integration, patient engagement and adherence, health behavior change, and new technologies in diagnosis and treatment. Prior to Happify, he was senior medical director of New Product and Innovation for Optum, where he spearheaded the formation of a telebehavioral service and was part of the team bringing innovation to this sector. Previously he served as Optum's western regional medical director and medical director for Tricare–Western

Region with Health Net, where he gained experience with large government contracts and coordinated with the VA and DoD. Murray received his BA from the University of Pennsylvania, his MD from the University of Rochester, and completed his psychiatric residency at UCLA.

Megan Zweig

Megan Zweig is chief operating officer of Rock Health, an early-stage digital health venture fund and advisory services firm with headquarters in San Francisco. Rock Health states that it is the first venture fund dedicated to digital health. Its large and growing portfolio includes some of the most innovative healthcare companies in segments that include dental benefits management, telehealth, HIPAA compliance, pediatric care management, predictive analytics, and prescription and pharmaceuticals management.

As Chief Operating Officer, Megan leads the Enterprise Membership, research, and operations teams at Rock Health. Through thought partnership, the power of community, and market-leading research, her teams support enterprise clients advancing their digital health strategies via the startup innovation ecosystem. Prior to joining Rock Health, Megan worked at The Advisory Board Company, where she led the Physician Executive Council, an organization that supports chief medical officers at more than 1,300 hospitals and health systems nationwide. Megan received an MBA from Berkeley Haas, where she graduated valedictorian of her executive MBA class in January 2020. Megan graduated cum laude from Duke University, earning a BA in public policy studies with a focus on health policy.

INDEX